SHARON RAINEY

the
Best Part
of
My Day

Healing ✳ Journal

CarePath Publications

Copyright ©2016 by Sharon E. Rainey

All rights reserved.

The Best Part of My Day - Healing Journal

by Sharon E. Rainey

ISBN 978-0-9830868-1-9

Design by J.A. Creative

CarePath Publications

1146-D Walker Road, Great Falls, VA 22066

www.carepathpublications.com

First printing October 2016

NOTICE OF LIABILITY

The author has made every effort to check and ensure the accuracy of the information presented in this book. However, the information herein is sold without warranty, either expressed or implied. Neither the author, publisher, nor any dealer or distributor of this book will be held liable for any damages caused indirectly or directly by the information contained in this book.

DISCLAIMER

The author and publisher are not engaged in rendering medical or psychological services. Every effort has been made to provide the most up to date and accurate information possible. Technological changes may occur at any time after the publication of this book. This book may contain typographical and content errors; therefore this is only designed as a guide and a resource.

TO MY HUSBAND JEFFREY

Each moment with you is the best part of my day

Each laugh, each smile, each whisper

I love you to infinity and beyond

TO OUR SON STEPHEN

Our love for you is steadfast, deep, infinite

Here is to your journey of finding

The Best Part of Your Day

Table of Contents

How "The Best Part of My Day" Started

When our son Stephen got into the car from elementary school each day, he was quick to tell me the worst part of his day. It often involved another student making fun of him or someone breaking the class rules. Stephen was an ardent rule-follower, so when someone else broke the rules, it was disturbing to him.

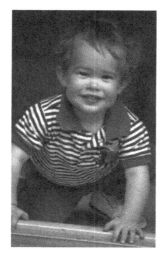

It was difficult for Stephen to see what had gone well in the day. His early life was filled with surgery, medical procedures and frequent hospitalizations. He had dealt with more life-critical issues than most middle-aged men.

But as a sufferer of depression for many years, I knew the importance of trying to find positive experiences in each day, no matter how small. I didn't know how to 'teach' this to Stephen, but I realized it was an important element in his development.

OUR SON, STEPHEN

I started asking Stephen, "What was the BEST part of your day?" He would think hard with the initial answers usually being "lunch" or "recess". When I started ruling those options out, he looked more closely at his interactions with others. And he started finding more "best parts" of his day. Some days were more of a struggle than others, but I think he caught on and realized that focusing on the positive can impact one's perspective in a dramatic way at times.

When Stephen was six years old, we spent a week of summer vacation in Williamsburg, Virginia. It was hot, muggy, crowded, and exhausting. My husband Jeffrey is a contractor with an extensive background in historic restoration, and this trip was a way to show his son some of what he used to do. At the end of the trip as we started home, we asked Stephen, "What was the best part of the trip?" Jeff was hoping for something like the brickmaking, barrel making, silver-smithing.

"Running down the middle of the road catching raindrops on my tongue," Stephen instantly replied, smiling large. That reply, with the wide smile on his face, is a precious memory I carry to this day. Sometimes, we won't know what the best part is for someone else; it is a great discussion to initiate.

Now, it is a family custom to talk about the best part of our respective days, whether we were all doing our own thing in different places or were together for an event or adventure.

Developing
The Idea

In 2009, I started treatment for co-infections of Lyme disease. I had been sick for 30 years off and on without a clear diagnosis. Admittedly, by this time, I was depressed. It was hard to find anything positive in my life except that I had finally found a physician who understood what was wrong with me and was treating my disease effectively.

Part of that treatment included ingesting drugs that made me feel worse for a few days and then, ever so slightly, I would improve. It was the "3 steps forward, 2.5 steps backward" routine. Throughout treatment for the first two and a half years, there were days and weeks that were absolutely miserable. By miserable, I mean I couldn't get out of bed unless it was to the bathroom and even that felt as though I was in a marathon. Joint pain, deep bone pain, brain fog, the inability to write a note or read a book – day after day. It was difficult to maintain hope.

Stephen came home and asked me how my day was and I immediately went to the worst of my day. With a small grin on his face, he asked, "Well, then, what was the BEST part of your day?"

The student had become the teacher.

In that instant, I realized that if I focused on the pain and misery, it would take me longer to heal. I needed to figure out a way to focus on the positive moments of each day. I needed to see where I was improving and healing. But when chronic pain is my most often companion, it can be challenging to keep looking for the good.

What Counts and What Doesn't

On my birthday in 2014, I didn't do anything in particular. The best part of my day was eating a Mexican lunch with my husband and two employees. It was a delicious lunch, but the best part was the time we spent together laughing, talking, and connecting. It was casual, comfortable and ordinary.

Two days later, I watched my husband Jeffrey endure a heart attack in the emergency room of our local hospital. I wasn't sure he would survive as I watched his blood pressure soar to 213/175. His genetic history was not a promising factor with both sides of his family riddled with heart attacks starting at age 50. Jeff was 58.

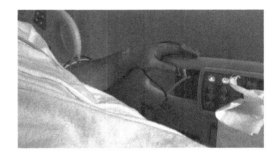

That morning, Jeff had woken up with a nagging cough. He arrived at the doctor's office at 9 am, dismissed 20 minutes later with a prescription for cough medicine. Another thirty minutes later, we were in the emergency room listening to the doctor describe a possible pulmonary embolism. Two hours after that, another physician told us Jeffrey had a heart attack. Then we heard it was a heart attack and a possible blood clot. In the catheterization lab, the radiology cardiologist placed four stents, three of which are in the "widow-maker" artery, and a warning that open-heart surgery was not yet ruled out.

Throughout the entire crisis, weirdly enough, I was the calm one. Let me rephrase that. AFTER I watched him have the heart attack, with his blood pressure up at 213/175, and thinking he would die at that very moment, AFTER that, I was overcome with the most mysterious but completely grounded confirmation that everything was going to be ok.

I took each hour of the crisis as it came, looking no further. I was calm, reassuring, and even trying to make Jeffrey laugh. Jeff didn't want any visitors so I politely refused friends' and families' offers to come to the hospital. Selfishly, I wanted to be alone with him. It wasn't that desperate "I need to be with you" feeling. It was that "I am so in love with you I can't imagine where else I would be right now" feeling. Again, in an instant, all the nonsense in life collapsed to the floor and all that mattered was the time I spent with Jeff, holding his hand, running my fingers through his hair, talking with him, laughing, and yes, even crying with him. Every moment during those days were (and remain) precious to me.

Heather, Jeff's daughter, came to visit the first night. She needed to see her dad, hug him and hold him. Even at 30-something, Heather was very frightened; rightfully so. Her father had escaped death. The second day, our son Stephen arrived from college and Heather returned.

The nursing staff, radiology techs, and even physicians wasted no time telling each of us why and how Jeffrey should not have survived this "cardiac event." They listed in detail each significant occurrence that should have caused death, and yet here he was, vibrantly alive. The ones willing to share their faith with us made it clear that God was controlling the outcome of Jeffrey's healing. Over and over, for two days and nights, we heard, "He really shouldn't be here. He is one lucky man."

Hearing this repeatedly gave us a clear view that this was a second chance and we ought not waste it. By this point, we were all tearful and grateful and still terrified. But being together sweetened this crisis. The time with Heather and Stephen, sharing our fear, relief and gratitude together, was a treasured moment that still bonds us.

Twenty years before, on a cold February afternoon, Jeff and I brought Stephen into our bedroom, sandwiched his newborn body between ours, and we watched him sleep. As his chest rose and fell, we knew our lives had changed forever. Jeff and I smiled with joy and anticipation, whispering, wondering what our son's new life would bring -- a little fear, but so much hope and so many dreams. This was especially sweet because Stephen had been born with a birth defect that required immediate surgery. He almost died two days after his surgery and spent another sixteen days in the Newborn Intensive Care Unit (NICU) in Children's Hospital. We almost lost the opportunity to bring our baby home to watch him sleep.

Two days after the heart attack started, Jeffrey was home, lying in bed next to me. I watched him sleep, just as when we brought Stephen home. I knew this was a new beginning for both of us. In a sense, Jeffrey was starting again. Again, some fear, but more so, hope and dreams abounded.

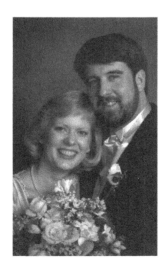

JEFF AND SHARON ON WEDDING DAY (1991)

I realized that every moment, every single moment I have with Jeffrey... *that* is the best part of my day. It is the moment when our love is tangibly connected profoundly taking deeper root than ever before in our previous 25 years together. This love I have for Jeffrey is further reaching, deeper, and more deeply rooted than ever.

Sounds cliché-ish, doesn't it? It might be, but it's what is true for me. I am married to my best friend, my soul mate, the man who makes me laugh every day. Every day Jeffrey tells me he loves me; he wants me. And he means it. His actions reinforce his words to me. When we hold hands together in the middle of the night, I know his love is deeper than ever before.

But we didn't always feel that way.

Jeffrey and I experienced many trials through 25 years of marriage: almost losing a child, polar opposite parenting styles, chronic illness, life threatening illnesses for our parents, death of a nephew by suicide, Jeff's father's death, my father's death, economic recession, challenges of both owning our own businesses. These obstacles are covered in more detail in my book *Lyme Savvy: Treatment Insights for Lyme Patients and Practitioners*. But through each trial has come triumph. And more love. Through each crisis, we have come back to the two of us – our relationship. We remain determined to build our love and to let that love rule above everything else.

Love Wins

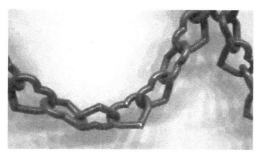

PHOTO BY STEPHEN RAINEY

In *365 Prescriptions for the Soul,* Dr. Bernie Siegel writes: "The greatest truth I know about life is that love is the answer. If you ask me what the question is, I will tell you it is every question you could ever ask. Love is always the answer to every question and problem. We are here to love and be loved and learn a few things in the process. I can never be wrong when I choose to love. Love rewards me by bringing meaning to my life."

For me, I had to take it one step further. Sometimes, the answer isn't always enough.

About 20 years ago, a friend recommended a new author to me (no, I am not going to tell you who it is). This author wrote some romance books but also mysteries. I read two of her books and loved them -- just my style, attention span, etc. The third book, a mystery, however, was disturbing. As in, I couldn't sleep when I finished. In the last paragraph of the book, the villain rode out of town on the train. Evil had not been conquered – it had merely been chased out of town.

A few years earlier, I left a bad first marriage that had originally taken me half way around the world, isolating me from friends and family, and filling me with fear and doubt.

When I left that marriage, I left the insanity, the indifference, the negativity.

In my world, LOVE MUST WIN. It can't just be the answer. It must conquer all evil, all hatred, all indifference.

Yes, Love is the always the answer, no matter the question. But Love always wins. Love always conquers (if we allow it).

When we have loved, that loving part is the best part of any and every day.

Sometimes the best part of the day is merely realizing that love wins and seeing it actualized in the day's events.

When I am in a difficult situation, especially when it involves another person, I can feel "stuck" on what I should do or say or think.

The simplest resolution for me in such circumstances has been to answer the following question, **"What is the next right thing to do (or say, or not say)?"**

And when I cannot clearly answer that, I then ask, **"What is the next most loving thing I can do (or say, or not say)?"**

Asking these two questions has exponentially simplified my life and expanded my feeling of love and fulfillment. And while it may sound simple, I acknowledge that it is not always easy. But it is so worth doing.

How the Idea Became Tangible

Throughout my chronic illness (co-infections of Lyme Disease) and healing journey, I had trouble maintaining focus and keeping what little energy I had in moving forward. I had days when I could find nothing positive. I had trouble remembering to take my meds, or even to eat.

When I didn't feel good, I was openly critical of myself and of those around me. It wasn't much fun to be around the sick one (me). I had to find a way to get myself out of the negativity. I had to take responsibility for my healing.

Throughout treatment, my physician asked me to make some significant daily changes in my life. He explained that if I chose not to make those changes, my chances for complete healing were seriously compromised. But trying to change everything all at once was often confusing and frustrating and entirely overwhelming. Being self-critical was one of those habits he said I needed to break.

My physician is a man who likes "data." He looks at trends. He wanted to know "on average" how many hours a night I was sleeping, how often I was taking all my medication, what healthy foods I was taking in.

It is hard for me to see trends. I get "mired in the weeds." The only way I could figure out how to keep track was to create a spreadsheet. Eventually, I wanted to see if I could graph the data and get that "big picture" scene. The first spreadsheet was just a running list of accomplishments. I recorded the task and the date. For instance:

DATE	TASK
June 19, 20XX	Unloaded the top half of the dishwasher
September 3, 20XX	Made the bed in the morning
November 30, 20XX	Wore make up to work again.

I also recorded when I started new major meds in the treatment protocol so that if I was taking a few too many steps backward, I could remind myself why that was happening.

When that became easier to complete, I took the next step of trying to keep track of other tasks. I started a spreadsheet that was more of a checklist to make sure I was doing what I needed to do on a daily basis.

DATE	1/14/15	1/15/15	1/16/15
MEDS	7	6	7
DETOX	Lemon water	Epsom Salt	Dry brushing
GREEN SMOOTHIE	Yes	No	No
APPLE CIDER VINEGAR	Yes	Yes	Yes
VITAMIN C POWDER	No	No	No
WALK	No	No	No
REST/NAP	Nap	Rest	Rest
MEDITATE/ PRAY	No	Yes	Yes

This chart can be about anything. These were the things I was having trouble staying consistent with. In the meds column, I was supposed to take meds 7 times each day. I didn't always take each dose, so that column would tell the doctor I was being maybe 80% compliant with all my meds. Some days I didn't need to detox from therapy, so it might be blank. Filling in a chart was simple for me.

What Helps
Us Heal

As I began to feel considerably better, I evaluated which elements of my healing were the most significant. Obviously, following the doctor's protocol was a major component. Taking my meds was important. But I wanted to delve deeper. Many patients take the meds and follow doctors' orders, but they don't necessarily heal. I was trying to figure out what made my journey different from theirs'.

It was in this study that I realized it's not just about taking the meds. While some of this may vary for each person, I do think there are common base elements essential for anyone dealing with a chronic illness to be able to heal. I believe those include:

- therapeutic rest
- laughter
- helping others / getting outside of your head
- feeling joy
- nourishing one's body, mind, and soul
- prayer and meditation
- offering kindness to others and receiving kindness from others
- forgiveness
- gratitude

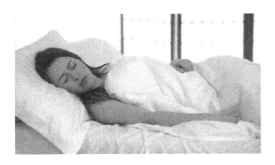

THERAPEUTIC REST

With Lyme Disease or any other chronic/major illness, rest is critical in healing. To give the body a chance to recover, lying in bed with my head level with my heart was a decisive part of healing. And I had to do that every day. Complete rest was important. When I say rest, I mean TOTAL rest. Not just sitting on the sofa and watching

TV. I mean lying on the bed, my heart level with my head. The heart doesn't have to work nearly as hard in this position. I often viewed myself as being lazy when I was lying down. My husband was taking care of chores, cooking dinner, running errands. And I was lying on the bed. It took a lot of self-talk, a lot of talking with Jeff, and a lot of talking with my physician about the true need for deep rest and deep sleep. Because if I was resting and feeling guilty or having negative thoughts, I wasn't truly in a healing mode.

Insomnia is often an issue for chronically ill patients. Keeping track of how much sleep and/or rest I got was important for me. When I was so 'tired,' it was often because I had not slept well the previous three nights. To see it on paper made it more objective, less subjective (and therefore less emotional and judgmental). I could take the information, using it to change the direction I was headed in. Instead of beating myself up for not sleeping, I could justify the need for a long nap that next afternoon. No more martyring myself.

When I was pregnant with Stephen, I went into pre-term labor at 29 weeks. I spent ten weeks in bed while taking Terbutaline. I call Terbutaline 'the drug from hell' because it made my hands shaky. I couldn't read or do needlepoint. I couldn't write. I couldn't focus enough even to watch a television show. I was angry I had to take the drug and that I had to be in bed. A friend reminded me I needed to focus on the baby.

"Today, you are helping to create a kidney," Anne would say. Each week we read the process of development in a child and I would focus on those, knowing that my resting and obeying doctor's orders were helping to create this child as a whole.

When lying in bed during medical treatment, I became restless and frustrated. I started feeling sorry for myself. So I started visualizing my cells healing and becoming the shapes they should be. I had seen healthy blood smears and my own blood smears. I knew what to aim for. I imagined the cells healthy and filled with nutrients.

LAUGHTER

Laughter is critical to healing. This realization came to me after our nephew's suicide. I cried and cried and cried. I couldn't seem to run out of the tears. So I started watching the bloopers from "Whose Line is it Anyway" on YouTube. I watched at least 30 minutes each day. Laughing for those 30 minutes didn't absolve my grief, but it made getting up each day a little easier. When I could find something to laugh about, my grief lightened just enough to make the day bearable.

It also became easier to laugh in other situations once I could laugh at the TV. I could laugh in a conversation or laugh in a situation that previously might have caused me to tear up. Laughter lightens my heart and therefore heals my soul as well. And with the gift of the Internet these days, it's pretty easy to find something to laugh with and enjoy. I'm also a "Big Bang Theory" fan. Anything that makes you laugh is good.

GIVING IT AWAY

When I feel exhausted and depressed, I also often feel sorry for myself. That is a dangerous place for me to be. That's a signal for me that I need to DO something. But when fatigue is this strong, it's often hard to find the 'something' that I am capable of doing.

This is essential for my healing. I have to help others. Initially, it was simply writing a note to a fellow Lyme patient or to a friend I hadn't seen in some time. It doesn't have to be big. It just needs to be something.

I listened to a friend sob over the phone one day for about 15 minutes. I couldn't fix her pain. But I could be a safe outlet for her to vent. A year later, that same friend paid the favor back to me.

I meet other newly diagnosed patients for coffee, offering them my own experience, strength and hope. I can't cure anyone. I can't guarantee they will heal. I can only tell them my story, remind them that they are not alone in their journey and offer a glimmer of hope for healing.

The key element to the success of this is that **it is important to help others without any detriment to yourself.** If you are choosing to help others without keeping your own health as your number one priority, then you are self-sabotaging and are only headed for more illness.

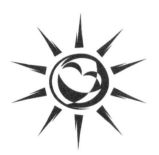

JOY

Early in my healing from Lyme Disease, I dramatically reduced my activity level and number of interactions with others. I stopped going out after 5 pm and I reduced my weekend activities to just one activity per weekend. Sounds pretty harsh, but it worked for me. Every single activity I chose to do was based on two questions:

1. Will this help me heal?
2. Will this bring me joy?

Obviously, doing the laundry doesn't qualify in this category. But going to the movies with my husband, meeting our son for dinner, and having coffee with a friend are all items that might encourage my body, mind and soul to move in a positive direction.

These two questions also made it easier for me to weed out my fair weather friends. It made it easier for me to say "No" when asked to volunteer or do something I might have said yes to previously.

And just to let you know, in case someone else hasn't told you yet: "NO" is a complete sentence. It does not require an explanation to follow. You can truly answer someone's request with a simple No. Try it. It will start to become easier each time you say it.

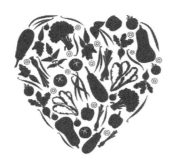

NOURISHMENT

Putting the right foods into my body helped me heal. And yes, I wasn't always (and still am not) the best at the diet changes. As part of my healing journey, I did start eating organic foods, consuming more fresh vegetables, drinking green smoothies and apple cider vinegar (not together!), eliminating dairy, soy, and gluten from my diet. Sugar is an addiction I still fight on a daily basis. And yes, I am well aware that sugar feeds bacteria in my body.

I am obese, so this is a sensitive topic for me. I added weight during my pregnancy, then doubled it with antidepressants (thanks, Paxil). Peripheral neuropathy, DVTs (blood clots), menopause, low thyroid and adrenal function also complicate the process of losing weight.

I share this with you because I tend to criticize myself very harshly about what I put in my mouth. I had to figure out a way to see this in a positive light. So I started recording what I did that nourished my body. That seems to help.

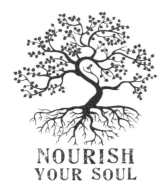

I also started recording what I did to nourish my mind. For me, most of the time, that nourishment comes in the form of writing or reading. It was important for me to focus on the positive actions taken to heal instead of beating myself up over what I did wrong each day. It shifts my perspective, thus making my body and mind more hospitable places for healing and positive energy.

Nourishing my soul occurred more subtly. And sometimes it came in weird packages. Nourishing my soul includes lunch or coffee with a friend, a card in the mail, watching and hearing a child laugh. It can be listening to the wind on an autumn afternoon or soaking the sun in at the end of the day. It can be a meeting I attended – a phone call with my parents. But I have found that when my soul feels nourishment, joy has also been involved in the experience as well. And laughter pops in there a time or two as well.

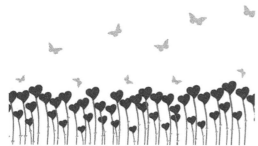

PRAYER AND MEDITATION

For some people, this may be a difficult step. And for most people, it's very personal.

During treatment for Lyme Disease, at my second appointment with my physician, he asked how my meditation and prayer were going.

"What?" I asked incredulously. I WANTED to say, "Who the hell are you to ask me about that?" I was completely surprised, caught off guard.

"Time for quiet thought is a very important element of your healing," he suggested quietly (and sternly). "It gives you space to talk to your Higher Power and more importantly, sometimes, to listen to that Higher Power."

This man knew more about healing than I did. I needed to listen to his insight, internalize it, and put it into action.

I pray, but meditation is more difficult for me. Deepak Chopra once said that he is up by 4 am each day to spend at least two hours in a meditative state. Yeah, no, that's not me. But I try to make meditation a part of my daily habits. Even if it is ten minutes, it is a time for me to practice listening and being open to possibilities that I might not have previously even noticed.

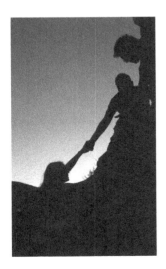

OFFERING KINDNESS AND ACCEPTING KINDNESS FROM OTHERS

Offering Kindness — When we offer a kindness to someone else, it helps us get outside of ourselves, but more importantly, it incorporates compassion into our daily lives. It's "easy" to do someone a favor. It takes a different thought process to offer a kindness to another individual.

First, I have to find an opportunity to provide that kindness, which means I'm keeping an eye open most of the day, looking outside of myself. When I offer that kindness, it is best when we can do such things anonymously so the ego stays out of play.

Accepting Kindness – In my experience, I have found this task to be more difficult. It has always been easier for me to give to others. It has been more problematic to accept help from others. The challenge for many of us, in accepting kindness from others, is to believe we are worthy of such acts. And that is precisely why it is so important in our healing to do just that: believe and accept that we are worthy of others' kindnesses bestowed upon us. We don't have to go looking for someone to "be nice" to us. This task is simply to affirm when others have offered us such, to affirm our worthiness in our world.

FORGIVENESS

Some readers are probably already cringing at this section. But forgiveness is HUGE in healing. Hang in there with me for a minute or two. Let's break this into two types of forgiveness.

LETTING THEM OFF THE HOOK FORGIVENESS

Every day, someone does something somewhere that annoys us. It can be the person who steals our parking spot, the bank teller who is short tempered, the grocery clerk that moves too slowly, the barista who gets our order wrong. It can be someone who says, "When are you going to be well?" or "Why aren't you better yet?" or the old favorite, "But you don't look sick." It can be the driver who almost hit my car, or the child who won't stop whining.

We can choose to hold onto that anger, that annoyance, that righteous indignation. Or, each day, we can choose one person and say, "Ok, I'm going to let you off the hook today for no reason other than for my own sanity and happiness." It's actually pretty cool to do. It can almost become a game. Try it for a few days and see what happens internally for you.

You are not required to actually say those words to that person out loud. You can say it within yourself and then record that you just did! Remember, this is something to help you heal, not something to start an argument with.

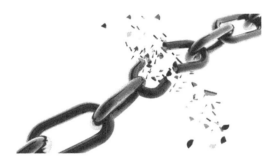

BIG FORGIVENESS.

I won't dilly-dally around on this topic.

I was a victim of sexual abuse by a Methodist minister. I know about trauma, about anger, about all that stuff that is painful, ugly and consuming. I also know what remaining a victim can do to a person's soul. I know what it did to mine. I had every right to be angry, resentful, and vengeful. I wanted him to hurt as much as he hurt me. It took me decades to acknowledge his abuse for what it was. And to have that abuse compounded with having my trust broken by someone supposedly in the healing profession was a two-tiered betrayal and injury.

I prayed to God to help me walk through this pain and to teach me, show me how to forgive one of His servants for his sins against a vulnerable child. Little by little, I saw or heard messages that helped me see how my holding onto this pain was doing me no favors whatsoever.

After listening to my anger and complaining in a meeting, a friend, John Agnew, leaned across the table, took off his glasses and asked, "Well, what do you want? You have to decide what you want. Do you want to be RIGHT? Or do you want to be HAPPY? And you may not choose both. It's one or the other."

I was stunned. Flabbergasted actually. It took me months to make my decision. I wanted the minister to admit to his bad deeds, to admit that I was certainly not the only one. I wanted him to admit if he had molested his daughter. I wanted him to be held accountable for every bad thing he had ever done to every innocent child. I wanted him to admit in public what he had done to me. I wanted him to accept responsibility for the pain he caused in so many aspects of my life. I wanted his career to be ruined. I wanted the entire community to know what this man had done to me and to others. And I knew I would never get any of that.

So I decided I wanted to be happy. I decided God would take care of His servants. I decided that when I went to Heaven, I knew I would be allowed in and that I need not worry about anybody else. I knew my healing would commence upon the cessation of my obsession with this minister's public persona. It was none of my business what happened to him. Eventually, he would answer to God for his doings. But in the meanwhile, I didn't need to endure any more suffering. I could "let go and let God" do His work.

My first marriage was to an emotionally unstable man who stalked me and threatened me before any stalking laws existed. I was alone in a foreign country trying to get back to the US. I feared for my life, my wellbeing. I feared he would utilize the skills he had learned in his line of work. I had bodyguards for several months after my attorney received threatening phone calls during the divorce process.

I prayed to God to help heal the first husband. I asked Him to heal B., to give B all the things in life and love that God thought he should have. I asked God to bring light and love into B's life so that he could heal and become the person that God wanted him to be. I don't know if that ever happened, but I still pray for him every day, that God gives him all that He wants for him to be happy and kind to those around him.

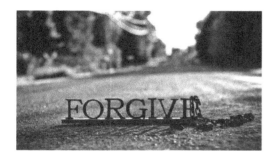

I know forgiveness is HARD. I know it is a process; that it doesn't come like a yes/no answer. I KNOW the pain, the fear, the anger, the bewilderment, the disconnecting. I KNOW the depersonalization, the wallowing. I know it. I was there numerous times, after numerous events, for more than a decade or two. **Extreme emotional pain has a profound effect on the body.** I witnessed my already frail body become even more toxic and plundered.

And I know the importance of letting it all go. I know that when I take that justifiable anger, the righteous indignation, the pain – when I take it back, I am not in a healing mode. **I have learned through repeated experiences that in order to heal, I MUST forgive.**

The forgiveness is <u>not</u> for the transgressor. The forgiveness is for **ME**.

Forgiveness does not mean that I approve of what happened. It does not mean I condone it.

Let me repeat here so you see it in case you missed it the first time.

Forgiveness does not mean I approve of or condone what transpired.

It took me a long, long time to fully grasp this.

The Aramaic word for "forgive" means literally to "untie." The fastest way to free the self from an enemy and all associated negativity is to forgive.

Untie those bindings; free yourself from that person's ugliness.

Hatred and anger had bound me to my pain.

Forgiveness enables me to walk away from that pain, the loneliness and suffering.

Forgiveness allows me to fulfill God's purpose, to love my imperfect self, to love others, and to be loved in healthy ways by positive individuals headed in the same direction with similar purpose.

GRATITUDE

So I just talked about doing some of the hardest things you have ever tried to do, including letting go of deep emotional pain.

And now I am asking you to go a step further. Now, I want you to find something to be grateful for – every single day.

Yep. I know – it sucks sometimes, doesn't it? But I wouldn't put this in here if it wasn't really necessary. I found out that by feeling grateful, by finding the good things in my life, however intricately miniscule they may be, I felt better. Not always a lot better – but better.

When we brought Stephen home from Children's Hospital the first time, I was grateful to have a child who survived. I met too many mothers in the breast pump room of the NICU who did not get to bring their child home. When we brought Stephen home from Children's Hospital the other times, I was grateful he was healing. And sometimes, I was just grateful it was sunny outside on the day he was released. I was grateful to come home to my own shower and bed.

When I thought Jeffrey was going to die during his heart attack, I kept giving thanks to God for the time I had been given with Jeff. Of course, I was pleading for God to let my husband live, but I was thankful for God bringing Jeff into my life for however long He desired us to be together.

When I sat with Jeff's dad in his final days, I was grateful to have the final chance to tell him everything I wanted him to know. I was grateful to be there as his soul transcended to heaven. It hurt like hell when he finally passed, but I was grateful to be a witness to the process and to be there as Jim let go of his loved ones here to be with his loved ones there. I was grateful that he was no longer in pain, no longer suffering with the many limitations his body had endured.

When my own father became terminally ill with only 26 days to live, I spent as many hours with him, not knowing how many we had left. I thanked him for the life he had given me. I told him all the important things he had taught me. I reminded him of all the things he had done and said that made me laugh. I promised him that my sisters and I would take care of Mom. I told him all that I admired in him. And when he asked me to write and give his eulogy, I did so with honor.

When I forgave the person who had run over my puppy and left him in the middle of the road, I was grateful for being able to remember the joy his Riley kisses gave me each morning and each night. I actually prayed for that person that s/he would find peace within. I hoped that s/he would find God's forgiveness and know that mine had already been given.

When I forgave the Methodist minister for his transgressions, I was grateful for the physical relief I felt as I let go of that last pound of pain.

Gratitude can be difficult. But it is essential to healing the body, the mind, and the soul. **We cannot fully heal if we cannot experience gratitude on a daily basis.**

Whew, that was heavy, wasn't it? Let's take a breather here; time to reflect on what was just covered.
At this point you are thinking that maybe this is a possibility for you OR you are thinking, "I'm just not there yet." That's ok.

It's where you are.

Healing is a process; it takes time. If you are not ready for the forgiveness or gratitude yet, let's just review the other things you can do to heal.

On a daily basis, you have the opportunities to:
- rest
- laugh
- help others
- feel joy
- nourish your body, mind, and soul
- pray and meditate
- offer kindness to others and
- accept kindness from others

Fulfill these opportunities on a daily basis. See what happens.

How This Book Developed into Its Present State

As the years passed, other chronically ill patients noticed my healing trend. They saw the difference. I was asked, "How do you do it?" almost daily. This isn't a magic potion. You don't try it one time and feel better.

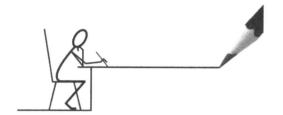

It is a process. It's a long process. It is a really, **really** long process. It is a process that requires daily practice and revision for the rest of my life. I am obligated to perform these tasks to STAY well.

I have to do them on my good days, my bad days, the days when my joints are too stiff to get out of bed, the days when my heart hurts for my children's and friends' troubled times.

I designed this book for me. I was tired of plain spreadsheets and jostled notes in my purse. I wanted one place to record it all - one place to glance through, remembering the best of the best. I wanted to acknowledge my good deeds and have a place to quickly and objectively record my healing actions.

And that's how I got to here, to sharing it with you. I hope you find it helpful, interesting, and positive. I hope it leads you to a path of healing and happiness.

Why the Quotes and the Question?

You will notice for each day, I include a quote and a question related to that quote. I have collected inspirational quotes for more than a decade. I find them encouraging and intriguing. The ones that have the most profound effect are often the ones I hear in conversations with friends or overhear in coffee shops amongst strangers. I even hear them in the doctors' offices' waiting rooms.

The quote and question are there for the nourishment of your soul. They are there to help you:

Grasp ⁙ **Acknowledge** ⁙ **Understand** ⁙ **Reach** ⁙ **Grow** ⁙ **Modify** ⁙ **Deepen** ⁙ **Solidify**

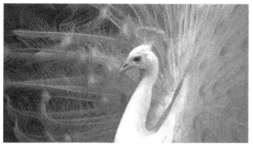

It is a way for you to help understand who you are, what you are. And more importantly, it is a way for you to accept and love your imperfect self as you are, right now, this moment, in this space.

We are not perfect beings. We were not designed that way. To continually try to achieve perfection in any form is not what our Higher Power wants for us. We are perfect in our imperfect form. We are exquisite souls housed in physical bodies. **We die in the negative energy. And we thrive with positive energy.**

Remember, Love Always Wins.

Love Always Conquers.

Love is always the answer, no matter the question.

When we have loved, that loving part is the best part of any and every day.

January 1ST

"It is healthier to see the good points of others than to analyze our own bad ones."
—FRANÇOISE SAGAN

Something good I saw in someone today: _____

The best part of my day: _____

Something that made me laugh: _____

Whom did I let "off the hook" today? _____

Someone / Something that brings me joy: _____

Where kindness touched my world today: _____

How I nourished my mind, body or spirit: _____

Number of hours I rested or slept in past 24 hours:
___ Rest   ___ Sleep

Prayer/Meditation for the day:
☼ Yes   ☼ No

I am grateful for: _____

Today I did this one little thing
For the earth...
for a friend or a stranger...
for someone older or younger...
for someone sicker...
in more need... _____

January 2ND

> *"If you can't change your fate, change your attitude."*
> —AMY TAN

Have I adjusted my attitude towards healing today? _____

The best part of my day: _____

Something that made me laugh: _____

Whom did I let "off the hook" today? _____

Someone / Something that brings me joy: _____

Where kindness touched my world today: _____

How I nourished my mind, body or spirit: _____

Number of hours I rested or slept in past 24 hours:
___ Rest ___ Sleep

Prayer/Meditation for the day:
☼ Yes   ☼ No

I am grateful for: _____

Today I did this one little thing
    For the earth...
        for a friend or a stranger...
            for someone older or younger...
                for someone sicker...
                    in more need... _____

January 3RD

> " *Everybody's heart is open when they have recently escaped from severe pain, or are recovering the blessing of health.* "
> —JANE AUSTEN

Something I am deserving of: _____

The best part of my day: _____

Something that made me laugh: _____

Whom did I let "off the hook" today? _____

Someone / Something that brings me joy: _____

Where kindness touched my world today: _____

How I nourished my mind, body or spirit: _____

Number of hours I rested or slept in past 24 hours:
___ Rest ___ Sleep

Prayer/Meditation for the day:
☼ Yes   ☼ No

I am grateful for: _____

Today I did this one little thing
    For the earth...
        for a friend or a stranger...
            for someone older or younger...
                for someone sicker...
                    in more need... _____

January 4TH

I am hopeful about: _____

The best part of my day: _____

Something that made me laugh: _____

Whom did I let "off the hook" today? _____

Someone / Something that brings me joy: _____

Where kindness touched my world today: _____

How I nourished my mind, body or spirit: _____

Number of hours I rested or slept in past 24 hours:
___ Rest ___ Sleep

Prayer/Meditation for the day:
☼ Yes ☼ No

I am grateful for: _____

Today I did this one little thing
    For the earth...
        for a friend or a stranger...
           for someone older or younger...
               for someone sicker...
                  in more need... _____

> **❝** *The pain of healing is far preferable to the pain of remaining at the effect of a neurotic pattern.* **❞**
> —MARIANNE WILLIAMSON

Am I experiencing the pain of healing today? _____

The best part of my day: _____

Something that made me laugh: _____

Whom did I let "off the hook" today? _____

Someone / Something that brings me joy: _____

Where kindness touched my world today: _____

How I nourished my mind, body or spirit: _____

Number of hours I rested or slept in past 24 hours:
____ Rest   ____ Sleep

Prayer/Meditation for the day:
☼ Yes   ☼ No

I am grateful for: _____

Today I did this one little thing
    For the earth...
        for a friend or a stranger...
            for someone older or younger...
                for someone sicker...
                    in more need... _____

January 6TH

"Where there is laughter there is always more health than sickness."
—PHYLLIS BOROME

Do I feel healthier today? If not,
how can I make myself feel healthier? _____

The best part of my day: _____

Something that made me laugh: _____

Whom did I let "off the hook" today? _____

Someone / Something that brings me joy: _____

Where kindness touched my world today: _____

How I nourished my mind, body or spirit: _____

Number of hours I rested or slept in past 24 hours:
___ Rest   ___ Sleep

Prayer/Meditation for the day:
☼ Yes   ☼ No

I am grateful for: _____

Today I did this one little thing
    For the earth...
        for a friend or a stranger...
            for someone older or younger...
                for someone sicker...
                    in more need... _____

> " *A further sign of health is that we don't become undone by fear and trembling, but we take it as a message that it is time to stop struggling and look directly at what is threatening us. Things like disappointment and anxiety are messengers telling us that we are about to go into unknown territory.* "

—PEMA CHODRON
WHEN THINGS FALL APART: HEART ADVICE FOR DIFFICULT TIMES

Something that nourished my soul: _____

The best part of my day: _____

Something that made me laugh: _____

Whom did I let "off the hook" today? _____

Someone / Something that brings me joy: _____

Where kindness touched my world today: _____

How I nourished my mind, body or spirit: _____

Number of hours I rested or slept in past 24 hours:
___ Rest ___ Sleep

Prayer/Meditation for the day:
☼ Yes ☼ No

I am grateful for: _____

Today I did this one little thing
    For the earth...
        for a friend or a stranger...
            for someone older or younger...
                for someone sicker...
                    in more need... _____

January 8TH

> *"What happened to you yesterday might not have been wonderful or even under your control. But who you become because of it, or in spite of it, is completely up to you."*
> —MARIANNE WILLIAMSON

I said yes to: _____

The best part of my day: _____

Something that made me laugh: _____

Whom did I let "off the hook" today? _____

Someone / Something that brings me joy: _____

Where kindness touched my world today: _____

How I nourished my mind, body or spirit: _____

Number of hours I rested or slept in past 24 hours:
___ Rest   ___ Sleep

Prayer/Meditation for the day:
☼ Yes   ☼ No

I am grateful for: _____

Today I did this one little thing
    For the earth...
        for a friend or a stranger...
            for someone older or younger...
                for someone sicker...
                    in more need... _____

"Climb inside this trust we've built. we've got walls to crash down, barriers to break thru, and entire universes to discover."

—TERRI ST. CLOUD
BONESIGHARTS.COM

Whom did I trust today? _____

The best part of my day: _____

Something that made me laugh: _____

Whom did I let "off the hook" today? _____

Someone / Something that brings me joy: _____

Where kindness touched my world today: _____

How I nourished my mind, body or spirit: _____

Number of hours I rested or slept in past 24 hours:
___ Rest   ___ Sleep

Prayer/Meditation for the day:
☼ Yes   ☼ No

I am grateful for: _____

Today I did this one little thing
    For the earth...
        for a friend or a stranger...
            for someone older or younger...
                for someone sicker...
                    in more need... _____

January 10TH

*"These physicians who treat chronic illness don't
just repair your body. They repair your soul."*
—UNKNOWN

How a professional has helped heal my soul: _____

The best part of my day: _____

Something that made me laugh: _____

Whom did I let "off the hook" today? _____

Someone / Something that brings me joy: _____

Where kindness touched my world today: _____

How I nourished my mind, body or spirit: _____

Number of hours I rested or slept in past 24 hours:
___ Rest   ___ Sleep

Prayer/Meditation for the day:
☼ Yes   ☼ No

I am grateful for: _____

Today I did this one little thing
    For the earth...
        for a friend or a stranger...
           for someone older or younger...
              for someone sicker...
                in more need... _____

Early Month Review

Best part of the past ten days? _____

Number of days I laughed: _____

Goal I want to set for the next 10 days: _____

Person/people who did or
said something to help me heal: _____

Anything else I have noticed
or want to remember/record: _____

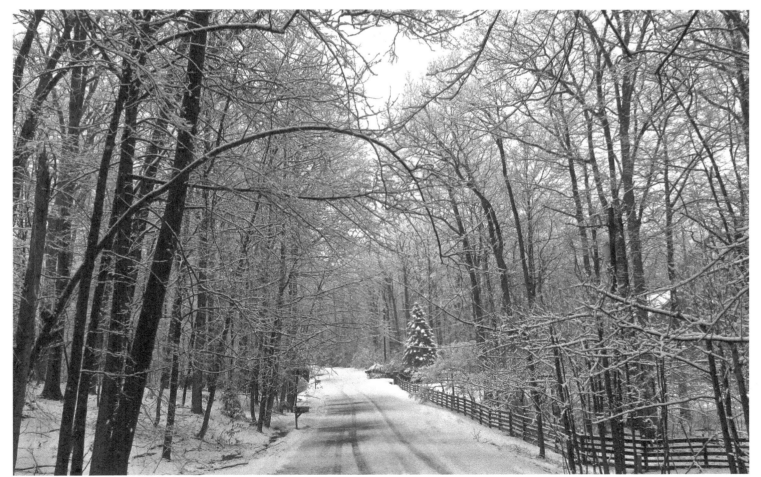

©NULLIE STOCKTON

January 11ᵀᴴ

> " *Forgiveness involves faith in a love that's greater than hatred, and a willingness to see the light in someone's soul even when their personality has harbored darkness. Forgiveness doesn't mean that someone didn't act horribly; it simply means that we choose not to focus on their guilt.* "
> —MARIANNE WILLIAMSON

I saw the light in _____ 's soul today.

The best part of my day: _____

Something that made me laugh: _____

Whom did I let "off the hook" today? _____

Someone / Something that brings me joy: _____

Where kindness touched my world today: _____

How I nourished my mind, body or spirit: _____

Number of hours I rested or slept in past 24 hours:
___Rest   ___Sleep

Prayer/Meditation for the day:
☼ Yes   ☼ No

I am grateful for: _____

Today I did this one little thing
    For the earth...
        for a friend or a stranger...
            for someone older or younger...
                for someone sicker...
                    in more need... _____

> " *Peace is not about being in a place where there is no trouble or hard work.*
> *It's about being in the midst of those things and still being calm in your heart.* "
> —ANONYMOUS

Something that calmed me today: _____

The best part of my day: _____

Something that made me laugh: _____

Whom did I let "off the hook" today? _____

Someone / Something that brings me joy: _____

Where kindness touched my world today: _____

How I nourished my mind, body or spirit: _____

Number of hours I rested or slept in past 24 hours:
___Rest   ___Sleep

Prayer/Meditation for the day:
☼ Yes   ☼ No

I am grateful for: _____

Today I did this one little thing
 For the earth...
   for a friend or a stranger...
     for someone older or younger...
       for someone sicker...
        in more need... _____

January 13TH

"I thought that it was expected of me to do what my family and friends thought I should do. I didn't really make decisions based on my true desires. Not completely anyways. I would get close to making my own decisions, but they would always be weak decisions, getting me a little closer to what I wanted but not quite getting there in full."

—ROBIN SHIRLEY
WWW.ROBINSHIRLEY.COM

One true desire I have: _____

The best part of my day: _____

Something that made me laugh: _____

Whom did I let "off the hook" today? _____

Someone / Something that brings me joy: _____

Where kindness touched my world today: _____

How I nourished my mind, body or spirit: _____

Number of hours I rested or slept in past 24 hours:
___ Rest   ___ Sleep

Prayer/Meditation for the day:
⋇ Yes   ⋇ No

I am grateful for: _____

Today I did this one little thing
    For the earth...
        for a friend or a stranger...
            for someone older or younger...
                for someone sicker...
                    in more need... _____

January 14TH

> *"If you admire greatness in another human being, it is your own greatness you are seeing."*
> —DEBBIE FORD

Where I saw greatness today: _____

The best part of my day: _____

Something that made me laugh: _____

Whom did I let "off the hook" today? _____

Someone / Something that brings me joy: _____

Where kindness touched my world today: _____

How I nourished my mind, body or spirit: _____

Number of hours I rested or slept in past 24 hours:
___ Rest ___ Sleep

Prayer/Meditation for the day:
☼ Yes ☼ No

I am grateful for: _____

Today I did this one little thing
    For the earth...
        for a friend or a stranger...
            for someone older or younger...
                for someone sicker...
                    in more need... _____

January 15TH

"Try to be like the turtle; at ease in your own shell."
—BILL COPELAND

Something about myself that I now accept: _____

The best part of my day: _____

Something that made me laugh: _____

Whom did I let "off the hook" today? _____

Someone / Something that brings me joy: _____

Where kindness touched my world today: _____

How I nourished my mind, body or spirit: _____

Number of hours I rested or slept in past 24 hours:
___ Rest ___ Sleep

Prayer/Meditation for the day:
☼ Yes ☼ No

I am grateful for: _____

Today I did this one little thing
For the earth...
for a friend or a stranger...
for someone older or younger...
for someone sicker...
in more need... _____

"Inhale, and God approaches you. Hold the inhalation, and God remains with you. Exhale, and you approach God. Hold the exhalation, and surrender to God."
—TIRUMALAI KRISHNAMACHARYA

Did I practice slow, deep breathing today? _____

The best part of my day: _____

Something that made me laugh: _____

Whom did I let "off the hook" today? _____

Someone / Something that brings me joy: _____

Where kindness touched my world today: _____

How I nourished my mind, body or spirit: _____

Number of hours I rested or slept in past 24 hours:
___ Rest   ___ Sleep

Prayer/Meditation for the day:
☼ Yes   ☼ No

I am grateful for: _____

Today I did this one little thing
    For the earth...
        for a friend or a stranger...
            for someone older or younger...
                for someone sicker...
                    in more need... _____

January 17TH

"If we take care of the moments, the years will take care of themselves."
—MARIA EDGEWORTH

A step I have taken today towards recovery: _____

The best part of my day: _____

Something that made me laugh: _____

Whom did I let "off the hook" today? _____

Someone / Something that brings me joy: _____

Where kindness touched my world today: _____

How I nourished my mind, body or spirit: _____

Number of hours I rested or slept in past 24 hours:
___ Rest   ___ Sleep

Prayer/Meditation for the day:
☼ Yes   ☼ No

I am grateful for: _____

Today I did this one little thing
    For the earth...
        for a friend or a stranger...
            for someone older or younger...
                for someone sicker...
                    in more need... _____

"*Greatness is the courage to overcome obstacles.*"
— DAVID HAWKINS, MD
LETTING GO: THE PATHWAY OF SURRENDER

I showed courage when I: _____

The best part of my day: _____

Something that made me laugh: _____

Whom did I let "off the hook" today? _____

Someone / Something that brings me joy: _____

Where kindness touched my world today: _____

How I nourished my mind, body or spirit: _____

Number of hours I rested or slept in past 24 hours:
___ Rest   ___ Sleep

Prayer/Meditation for the day:
☼ Yes   ☼ No

I am grateful for: _____

Today I did this one little thing
    For the earth...
        for a friend or a stranger...
            for someone older or younger...
                for someone sicker...
                    in more need... _____

January 19TH

> " *For each of us there is at least one place on the earth where our hearts and our bodies are mended and renewed. We need to find and go to these places if we are to learn how to dance... How can we recognize the places that teach us how to dance? By the way they let us sit still.* "
>
> —ORIAH MOUNTAIN DREAMER

(FROM HER BOOK THE DANCE ©2001, PUBLISHED BY HARPERONE, SAN FRANCISCO. ALL RIGHTS RESERVED. PRESENTED WITH PERMISSION OF THE AUTHOR. WWW.ORIAH.ORG)

My favorite place to be still: _____

The best part of my day: _____

Something that made me laugh: _____

Whom did I let "off the hook" today? _____

Someone / Something that brings me joy: _____

Where kindness touched my world today: _____

How I nourished my mind, body or spirit: _____

Number of hours I rested or slept in past 24 hours:
___ Rest   ___ Sleep

Prayer/Meditation for the day:
☼ Yes   ☼ No

I am grateful for: _____

Today I did this one little thing
    For the earth...
        for a friend or a stranger...
            for someone older or younger...
                for someone sicker...
                    in more need... _____

"Dismiss whatever insults your own soul; and your very flesh shall be a great poem, and have the richest fluency, not only in its words, but in the silent lines of its lips and face, and between the lashes of your eyes, and in every motion and joint of your body."
— WALT WHITMAN

How did I show love today? _____

The best part of my day: _____

Something that made me laugh: _____

Whom did I let "off the hook" today? _____

Someone / Something that brings me joy: _____

Where kindness touched my world today: _____

How I nourished my mind, body or spirit: _____

Number of hours I rested or slept in past 24 hours:
___Rest ___Sleep

Prayer/Meditation for the day:
☼ Yes ☼ No

I am grateful for: _____

Today I did this one little thing
    For the earth...
        for a friend or a stranger...
            for someone older or younger...
                for someone sicker...
                    in more need... _____

Mid Month Review

Best part of the past ten days? _____

Number of days I laughed: _____

Goal I want to set for the next 10 days: _____

Person/people who did or
said something to help me heal: _____

Anything else I have noticed
or want to remember/record: _____

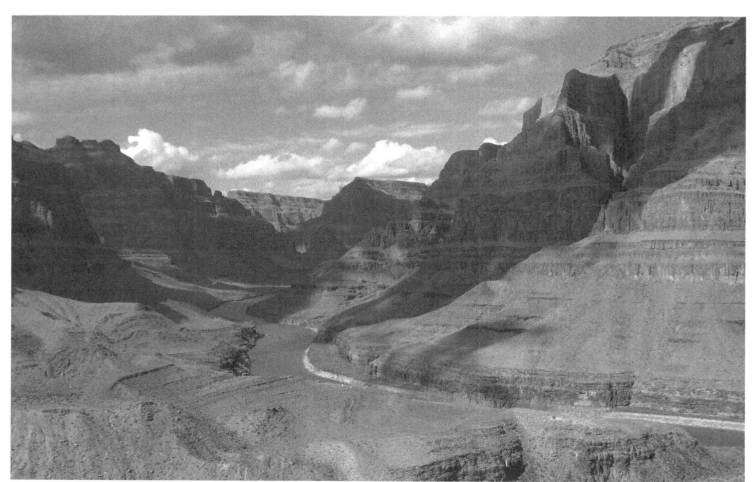

©CINDY MURPHY

> " *The truth is, laughter always sounds more perfect than weeping.*
> *Laughter flows in a violent riff and is effortlessly melodic. Weeping is*
> *often fought, choked, half strangled, or surrendered to with humiliation.* "
> —ANNE RICE

What laughter does for me: _____

The best part of my day: _____

Something that made me laugh: _____

Whom did I let "off the hook" today? _____

Someone / Something that brings me joy: _____

Where kindness touched my world today: _____

How I nourished my mind, body or spirit: _____

Number of hours I rested or slept in past 24 hours:
___ Rest   ___ Sleep

Prayer/Meditation for the day:
☼ Yes   ☼ No

I am grateful for: _____

Today I did this one little thing
    For the earth...
        for a friend or a stranger...
           for someone older or younger...
               for someone sicker...
                  in more need... _____

January 22ND

> "*Humor brings insight and tolerance.*"
> —AGNES REPPLIER

The brightest thing I saw today: _____

The best part of my day: _____

Something that made me laugh: _____

Whom did I let "off the hook" today? _____

Someone / Something that brings me joy: _____

Where kindness touched my world today: _____

How I nourished my mind, body or spirit: _____

Number of hours I rested or slept in past 24 hours:
___ Rest   ___ Sleep

Prayer/Meditation for the day:
☼ Yes   ☼ No

I am grateful for: _____

Today I did this one little thing
    For the earth...
        for a friend or a stranger...
            for someone older or younger...
                for someone sicker...
                    in more need... _____

"I must be willing to give up what I am in order to become what I will be."
—ALBERT EINSTEIN

I am willing to give up: _____

The best part of my day: _____

Something that made me laugh: _____

Whom did I let "off the hook" today? _____

Someone / Something that brings me joy: _____

Where kindness touched my world today: _____

How I nourished my mind, body or spirit: _____

Number of hours I rested or slept in past 24 hours:
___Rest   ___Sleep

Prayer/Meditation for the day:
☼ Yes   ☼ No

I am grateful for: _____

Today I did this one little thing
      For the earth...
            for a friend or a stranger...
                  for someone older or younger...
                        for someone sicker...
                              in more need... _____

January 24TH

"When I think about something, I invite it into my soul;
the more I think about it, the more welcome it makes itself."
—BARBARA BOYER

I invite… _____

The best part of my day: _____

Something that made me laugh: _____

Whom did I let "off the hook" today? _____

Someone / Something that brings me joy: _____

Where kindness touched my world today: _____

How I nourished my mind, body or spirit: _____

Number of hours I rested or slept in past 24 hours:
____Rest ____Sleep

Prayer/Meditation for the day:
☼ Yes ☼ No

I am grateful for: _____

Today I did this one little thing
    For the earth...
        for a friend or a stranger...
           for someone older or younger...
               for someone sicker...
                  in more need... _____

"If we had no winter, the spring would not be so pleasant; if we did not sometimes taste of adversity, prosperity would not be so welcome."
—ANNE BRADSTREET

I am trying to: _____

The best part of my day: _____

Something that made me laugh: _____

Whom did I let "off the hook" today? _____

Someone / Something that brings me joy: _____

Where kindness touched my world today: _____

How I nourished my mind, body or spirit: _____

Number of hours I rested or slept in past 24 hours:
___ Rest ___ Sleep

Prayer/Meditation for the day:
☼ Yes ☼ No

I am grateful for: _____

Today I did this one little thing
    For the earth...
        for a friend or a stranger...
            for someone older or younger...
                for someone sicker...
                    in more need... _____

January 26TH

*" The only meaningful thing we can offer one another is love. Not advice,
not questions about our choices, not suggestions for the future, just love. "*
—GLENNON DOYLE MELTON
(CARRY ON, WARRIOR: THE POWER OF EMBRACING YOUR MESSY, BEAUTIFUL LIFE)

How I showed love today: _____

The best part of my day: _____

Something that made me laugh: _____

Whom did I let "off the hook" today? _____

Someone / Something that brings me joy: _____

Where kindness touched my world today: _____

How I nourished my mind, body or spirit: _____

Number of hours I rested or slept in past 24 hours:
___ Rest   ___ Sleep

Prayer/Meditation for the day:
☀ Yes   ☀ No

I am grateful for: _____

Today I did this one little thing
    For the earth...
        for a friend or a stranger...
           for someone older or younger...
                for someone sicker...
                    in more need... _____

> **"** *If one advances confidently in the direction of his dreams, and endeavors to live the life which he has imagined, he will meet with success unexpected in common hours.* **"**
> —HENRY DAVID THOREAU

I feel confident about: _____

The best part of my day: _____

Something that made me laugh: _____

Whom did I let "off the hook" today? _____

Someone / Something that brings me joy: _____

Where kindness touched my world today: _____

How I nourished my mind, body or spirit: _____

Number of hours I rested or slept in past 24 hours:
___ Rest   ___ Sleep

Prayer/Meditation for the day:
☼ Yes   ☼ No

I am grateful for: _____

Today I did this one little thing
    For the earth...
        for a friend or a stranger...
            for someone older or younger...
                for someone sicker...
                    in more need... _____

January 28TH

" Tomorrow is the most important thing in life. Comes into us at midnight very clean. It's perfect when it arrives and it puts itself in our hands. It hopes we've learned something from yesterday. "
—JOHN WAYNE

What did I learn from yesterday? _____

The best part of my day: _____

Something that made me laugh: _____

Whom did I let "off the hook" today? _____

Someone / Something that brings me joy: _____

Where kindness touched my world today: _____

How I nourished my mind, body or spirit: _____

Number of hours I rested or slept in past 24 hours:
___ Rest   ___ Sleep

Prayer/Meditation for the day:
☼ Yes   ☼ No

I am grateful for: _____

Today I did this one little thing
    For the earth...
        for a friend or a stranger...
            for someone older or younger...
                for someone sicker...
                    in more need... _____

> *"In the depths of winter, I finally learned that there was in me an invincible summer."*
> —ALBERT CAMUS

How I am invincible: _____

The best part of my day: _____

Something that made me laugh: _____

Whom did I let "off the hook" today? _____

Someone / Something that brings me joy: _____

Where kindness touched my world today: _____

How I nourished my mind, body or spirit: _____

Number of hours I rested or slept in past 24 hours:
___ Rest   ___ Sleep

Prayer/Meditation for the day:
☀ Yes   ☀ No

I am grateful for: _____

Today I did this one little thing
    For the earth...
        for a friend or a stranger...
           for someone older or younger...
               for someone sicker...
                  in more need... _____

January 30TH

" I do not believe that sheer suffering teaches. If suffering alone taught, all the world would be wise, since everyone suffers. To suffering must be added mourning, understanding, patience, love, openness, and the willingness to remain vulnerable. "

—ANNE MORROW LINDBERGH

Am I willing to remain vulnerable
without remaining a victim? _____

The best part of my day: _____

Something that made me laugh: _____

Whom did I let "off the hook" today? _____

Someone / Something that brings me joy: _____

Where kindness touched my world today: _____

How I nourished my mind, body or spirit: _____

Number of hours I rested or slept in past 24 hours:
___ Rest   ___ Sleep

Prayer/Meditation for the day:
☼ Yes   ☼ No

I am grateful for: _____

Today I did this one little thing
    For the earth...
        for a friend or a stranger...
           for someone older or younger...
              for someone sicker...
                in more need... _____

> *"Perhaps God is even speaking to me in my tiredness
> and weariness about taking better care of myself."*
> —TREVOR HUDSON

Am I taking better care of myself today? _____

The best part of my day: _____

Something that made me laugh: _____

Whom did I let "off the hook" today? _____

Someone / Something that brings me joy: _____

Where kindness touched my world today: _____

How I nourished my mind, body or spirit: _____

Number of hours I rested or slept in past 24 hours:
___ Rest   ___ Sleep

Prayer/Meditation for the day:
☼ Yes   ☼ No

I am grateful for: _____

Today I did this one little thing
    For the earth...
        for a friend or a stranger...
           for someone older or younger...
               for someone sicker...
                  in more need... _____

End of Month Review

Best part of the past ten days? _____

Number of days I laughed: _____

Goal I want to set for the next 10 days: _____

Person/people who did or
said something to help me heal: _____

Anything else I have noticed
or want to remember/record: _____

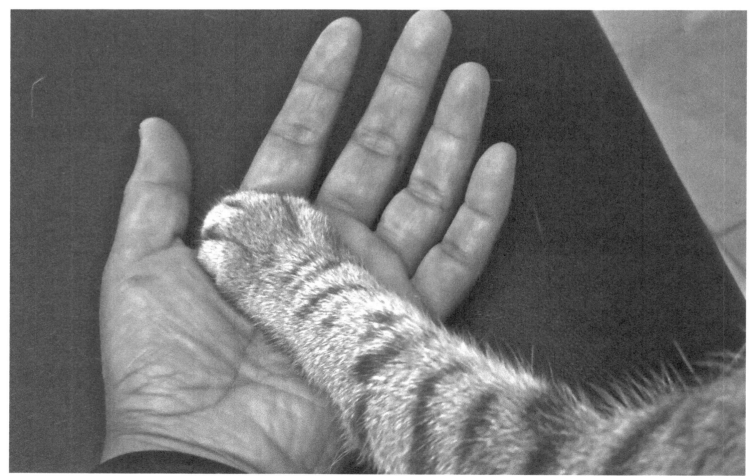

©NULLIE STOCKTON

> **"***You and you alone choose moment by moment***
> ***who and how you want to be in the world.***"**
>
> —JILL BOLTE TAYLOR
> *MY STROKE OF INSIGHT*

I am going to: _____

The best part of my day: _____

Something that made me laugh: _____

Whom did I let "off the hook" today? _____

Someone / Something that brings me joy: _____

Where kindness touched my world today: _____

How I nourished my mind, body or spirit: _____

Number of hours I rested or slept in past 24 hours:
____ Rest   ____ Sleep

Prayer/Meditation for the day:
☼ Yes   ☼ No

I am grateful for: _____

Today I did this one little thing
   For the earth...
      for a friend or a stranger...
         for someone older or younger...
           for someone sicker...
              in more need... _____

February 2ND

"*It's better to be alone than to have denial about your support structure.*"
—JENNIFER BOYKIN
WHEN PEOPLE DISAPPOINT. A LAMENT FOR THE "STRONG ONES.", OWNINGPINK.COM

Am I fully accepting of
what my support structure is? _____

The best part of my day: _____

Something that made me laugh: _____

Whom did I let "off the hook" today? _____

Someone / Something that brings me joy: _____

Where kindness touched my world today: _____

How I nourished my mind, body or spirit: _____

Number of hours I rested or slept in past 24 hours:
____ Rest   ____ Sleep

Prayer/Meditation for the day:
☼ Yes   ☼ No

I am grateful for: _____

Today I did this one little thing
    For the earth...
        for a friend or a stranger...
           for someone older or younger...
                for someone sicker...
                    in more need... _____

February 3RD

"He is happiest who hath power to gather wisdom from a flower."
—MARY HOWITT

Today I found wisdom in: _____

The best part of my day: _____

Something that made me laugh: _____

Whom did I let "off the hook" today? _____

Someone / Something that brings me joy: _____

Where kindness touched my world today: _____

How I nourished my mind, body or spirit: _____

Number of hours I rested or slept in past 24 hours:
___ Rest   ___ Sleep

Prayer/Meditation for the day:
☼ Yes   ☼ No

I am grateful for: _____

Today I did this one little thing
　　For the earth...
　　　　for a friend or a stranger...
　　　　　　for someone older or younger...
　　　　　　　　for someone sicker...
　　　　　　　　　　in more need... _____

February 4TH

"When something unexpected happens over which you have no control you must have the faith to trust that something greater than yourself will guide you."
—BETTY FORD

Is life filled with just coincidences
or something more? _____

The best part of my day: _____

Something that made me laugh: _____

Whom did I let "off the hook" today? _____

Someone / Something that brings me joy: _____

Where kindness touched my world today: _____

How I nourished my mind, body or spirit: _____

Number of hours I rested or slept in past 24 hours:
___ Rest   ___ Sleep

Prayer/Meditation for the day:
☼ Yes   ☼ No

I am grateful for: _____

Today I did this one little thing
    For the earth...
        for a friend or a stranger...
            for someone older or younger...
                for someone sicker...
                    in more need... _____

February 5TH

" We should all speak the words that we believe with our hearts. And stop speaking the words that we believe the world wants to hear from us. Say the things you have been wanting to say for years but never have. Do the things you have been dreaming of doing your whole life, but never have. Stop holding onto yourself so tightly. And your magic will be set free. "

—ROBIN SHIRLEY
WWW.ROBINSHIRLEY.COM

Today I say: _____

The best part of my day: _____

Something that made me laugh: _____

Whom did I let "off the hook" today? _____

Someone / Something that brings me joy: _____

Where kindness touched my world today: _____

How I nourished my mind, body or spirit: _____

Number of hours I rested or slept in past 24 hours:
___Rest ___Sleep

Prayer/Meditation for the day:
☼ Yes ☼ No

I am grateful for: _____

Today I did this one little thing
   For the earth...
      for a friend or a stranger...
         for someone older or younger...
           for someone sicker...
              in more need... _____

February 6ᵀᴴ

" *Waiting is one of the great arts.* "
—MARGERY ALLINGHAM

I am waiting for: _____

The best part of my day: _____

Something that made me laugh: _____

Whom did I let "off the hook" today? _____

Someone / Something that brings me joy: _____

Where kindness touched my world today: _____

How I nourished my mind, body or spirit: _____

Number of hours I rested or slept in past 24 hours:
___ Rest ___ Sleep

Prayer/Meditation for the day:
☀ Yes ☀ No

I am grateful for: _____

Today I did this one little thing
    For the earth...
        for a friend or a stranger...
           for someone older or younger...
              for someone sicker...
                in more need... _____

"If you think a complimentary thought about someone, don't just think it.
Dare to compliment people and pass on compliments to them from others."
—CATHERINE PONDER

A compliment I gave someone today: _____

The best part of my day: _____

Something that made me laugh: _____

Whom did I let "off the hook" today? _____

Someone / Something that brings me joy: _____

Where kindness touched my world today: _____

How I nourished my mind, body or spirit: _____

Number of hours I rested or slept in past 24 hours:
___ Rest   ___ Sleep

Prayer/Meditation for the day:
☼ Yes   ☼ No

I am grateful for: _____

Today I did this one little thing
   For the earth...
      for a friend or a stranger...
         for someone older or younger...
           for someone sicker...
              in more need... _____

February 8ᵀᴴ

"A gem cannot be polished without friction, nor a person perfected without trials."
—CHINESE PROVERB

A trial I overcame: _____

The best part of my day: _____

Something that made me laugh: _____

Whom did I let "off the hook" today? _____

Someone / Something that brings me joy: _____

Where kindness touched my world today: _____

How I nourished my mind, body or spirit: _____

Number of hours I rested or slept in past 24 hours:
___ Rest   ___ Sleep

Prayer/Meditation for the day:
☼ Yes   ☼ No

I am grateful for: _____

Today I did this one little thing
    For the earth...
        for a friend or a stranger...
           for someone older or younger...
              for someone sicker...
                in more need... _____

"I also think of reading as an act of faith, a hope I will discover something remarkable about ordinary life, about myself. And if the writer and the reader discover the same thing, if they have that connection, the act of faith has resulted in an act of magic."

—AMY TAN

An interesting article/book I read: _____

The best part of my day: _____

Something that made me laugh: _____

Whom did I let "off the hook" today? _____

Someone / Something that brings me joy: _____

Where kindness touched my world today: _____

How I nourished my mind, body or spirit: _____

Number of hours I rested or slept in past 24 hours:
____ Rest   ____ Sleep

Prayer/Meditation for the day:
☼ Yes   ☼ No

I am grateful for: _____

Today I did this one little thing
  For the earth...
      for a friend or a stranger...
          for someone older or younger...
              for someone sicker...
                  in more need... _____

February 10TH

" *The best way out of a problem is through it.* "
—ANONYMOUS

Something I am getting
through and not going around: _____

The best part of my day: _____

Something that made me laugh: _____

Whom did I let "off the hook" today? _____

Someone / Something that brings me joy: _____

Where kindness touched my world today: _____

How I nourished my mind, body or spirit: _____

Number of hours I rested or slept in past 24 hours:
___ Rest   ___ Sleep

Prayer/Meditation for the day:
☼ Yes   ☼ No

I am grateful for: _____

Today I did this one little thing
    For the earth...
        for a friend or a stranger...
           for someone older or younger...
              for someone sicker...
                in more need... _____

Early Month Review

Best part of the past ten days? _____

Number of days I laughed: _____

Goal I want to set for the next 10 days: _____

Person/people who did or
said something to help me heal: _____

Anything else I have noticed
or want to remember/record: _____

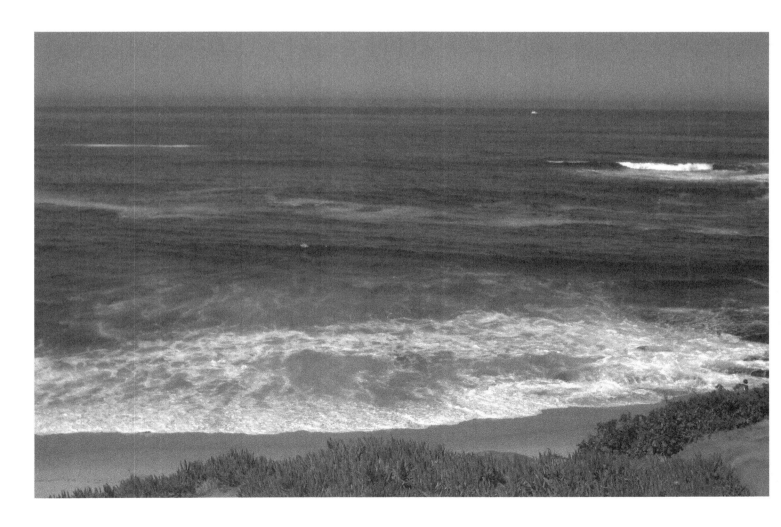

February 11TH

"It is the moment when I can hear, when I know, that an answer is being offered to me. All other sounds measurably fade, including the banter in my brain. It is when the answer travels from my heart to my head and says, "This is so." No questions follow, no objections interrupt; just the recognition that I must listen and follow."

—SHARON RAINEY
MAKING A PEARL FROM THE GRIT OF LIFE

What I heard today: _____

The best part of my day: _____

Something that made me laugh: _____

Whom did I let "off the hook" today? _____

Someone / Something that brings me joy: _____

Where kindness touched my world today: _____

How I nourished my mind, body or spirit: _____

Number of hours I rested or slept in past 24 hours:
___ Rest   ___ Sleep

Prayer/Meditation for the day:
☼ Yes   ☼ No

I am grateful for: _____

Today I did this one little thing
    For the earth...
        for a friend or a stranger...
            for someone older or younger...
                for someone sicker...
                    in more need... _____

" You must love and care for yourself, because that's when the best comes out."
—TINA TURNER

Something I did that shows
I love and care about myself: _____

The best part of my day: _____

Something that made me laugh: _____

Whom did I let "off the hook" today? _____

Someone / Something that brings me joy: _____

Where kindness touched my world today: _____

How I nourished my mind, body or spirit: _____

Number of hours I rested or slept in past 24 hours:
____ Rest   ____ Sleep

Prayer/Meditation for the day:
☼ Yes   ☼ No

I am grateful for: _____

Today I did this one little thing
    For the earth...
        for a friend or a stranger...
            for someone older or younger...
                for someone sicker...
                    in more need... _____

February 13TH

"What one loves in childhood stays in the heart forever."
—MARY JO PUTNEY

A favorite childhood memory: _____

The best part of my day: _____

Something that made me laugh: _____

Whom did I let "off the hook" today? _____

Someone / Something that brings me joy: _____

Where kindness touched my world today: _____

How I nourished my mind, body or spirit: _____

Number of hours I rested or slept in past 24 hours:
___ Rest   ___ Sleep

Prayer/Meditation for the day:
☼ Yes   ☼ No

I am grateful for: _____

Today I did this one little thing
    For the earth...
        for a friend or a stranger...
            for someone older or younger...
                for someone sicker...
                    in more need... _____

"Love from one being to another can only be that two solitudes
come nearer, recognize and protect and comfort each other."
—HAN SUYIN

Someone I said "I love you" to today: _____

The best part of my day: _____

Something that made me laugh: _____

Whom did I let "off the hook" today? _____

Someone / Something that brings me joy: _____

Where kindness touched my world today: _____

How I nourished my mind, body or spirit: _____

Number of hours I rested or slept in past 24 hours:
___ Rest ___ Sleep

Prayer/Meditation for the day:
☼ Yes ☼ No

I am grateful for: _____

Today I did this one little thing
   For the earth...
      for a friend or a stranger...
         for someone older or younger...
            for someone sicker...
               in more need... _____

February 15TH

" Reaching our limit is not some kind of punishment. It's actually a sign of health that, when we meet the place where we are about to die, we feel fear and trembling. A further sign of health is that we don't become undone by fear and trembling, but we take it as a message that it is time to stop struggling and look directly at what is threatening us. Things like disappointment and anxiety are messengers telling us that we are about to go into unknown territory."

—PEMA CHODRON

I listened to my body today by: _____

The best part of my day: _____

Something that made me laugh: _____

Whom did I let "off the hook" today? _____

Someone / Something that brings me joy: _____

Where kindness touched my world today: _____

How I nourished my mind, body or spirit: _____

Number of hours I rested or slept in past 24 hours:
___ Rest   ___ Sleep

Prayer/Meditation for the day:
☼ Yes   ☼ No

I am grateful for: _____

Today I did this one little thing
    For the earth...
        for a friend or a stranger...
            for someone older or younger...
                for someone sicker...
                    in more need... _____

"Enlightenment is not a process of learning, it is a process of unlearning."
—DR. KAT DOMINGO

Something I learned and unlearned today: _____

The best part of my day: _____

Something that made me laugh: _____

Whom did I let "off the hook" today? _____

Someone / Something that brings me joy: _____

Where kindness touched my world today: _____

How I nourished my mind, body or spirit: _____

Number of hours I rested or slept in past 24 hours:
___ Rest   ___ Sleep

Prayer/Meditation for the day:
☼ Yes   ☼ No

I am grateful for: _____

Today I did this one little thing
     For the earth...
          for a friend or a stranger...
               for someone older or younger...
                    for someone sicker...
                         in more need... _____

February 17TH

" Our children take away our time but they give us poems. "
—JESSE LEE KERCHEVEL

Something I learned from
watching or listening to a child: _____

The best part of my day: _____

Something that made me laugh: _____

Whom did I let "off the hook" today? _____

Someone / Something that brings me joy: _____

Where kindness touched my world today: _____

How I nourished my mind, body or spirit: _____

Number of hours I rested or slept in past 24 hours:
___ Rest   ___ Sleep

Prayer/Meditation for the day:
☼ Yes   ☼ No

I am grateful for: _____

Today I did this one little thing
    For the earth...
        for a friend or a stranger...
            for someone older or younger...
                for someone sicker...
                    in more need... _____

February 18TH

"We are just beginning to appreciate hope's reach and have not defined its limits. I see hope as the very heart of healing. For those who have hope, it may help some to live longer, and it will help all to live better."
—JEROME GROOPMAN

Do I want to be right or do I want to be happy? _____

The best part of my day: _____

Something that made me laugh: _____

Whom did I let "off the hook" today? _____

Someone / Something that brings me joy: _____

Where kindness touched my world today: _____

How I nourished my mind, body or spirit: _____

Number of hours I rested or slept in past 24 hours:
___ Rest   ___ Sleep

Prayer/Meditation for the day:
☼ Yes   ☼ No

I am grateful for: _____

Today I did this one little thing
    For the earth...
        for a friend or a stranger...
           for someone older or younger...
               for someone sicker...
                  in more need... _____

February 19TH

" Continuous effort — not strength or intelligence — is the key to unlocking our potential. "
—LIANE CORDES
THE REFLECTING POND: MEDITATIONS FOR SELF-DISCOVERY

How I am unlocking my potential: _____

The best part of my day: _____

Something that made me laugh: _____

Whom did I let "off the hook" today? _____

Someone / Something that brings me joy: _____

Where kindness touched my world today: _____

How I nourished my mind, body or spirit: _____

Number of hours I rested or slept in past 24 hours:
___Rest   ___Sleep

Prayer/Meditation for the day:
☼ Yes   ☼ No

I am grateful for: _____

Today I did this one little thing
    For the earth...
        for a friend or a stranger...
           for someone older or younger...
              for someone sicker...
                in more need... _____

" *Patience with others is Love, Patience with self is Hope, Patience with God is Faith.* **"**
—ADEL BESTAVROS

Something I heard, saw or did that
is an example of love, hope, or faith: _____

The best part of my day: _____

Something that made me laugh: _____

Whom did I let "off the hook" today? _____

Someone / Something that brings me joy: _____

Where kindness touched my world today: _____

How I nourished my mind, body or spirit: _____

Number of hours I rested or slept in past 24 hours:
___ Rest   ___ Sleep

Prayer/Meditation for the day:
☼ Yes   ☼ No

I am grateful for: _____

Today I did this one little thing
    For the earth...
        for a friend or a stranger...
            for someone older or younger...
                for someone sicker...
                    in more need... _____

Mid Month
Review

Best part of the past ten days? _____

Number of days I laughed: _____

Goal I want to set for the next 10 days: _____

Person/people who did or
said something to help me heal: _____

Anything else I have noticed
or want to remember/record: _____

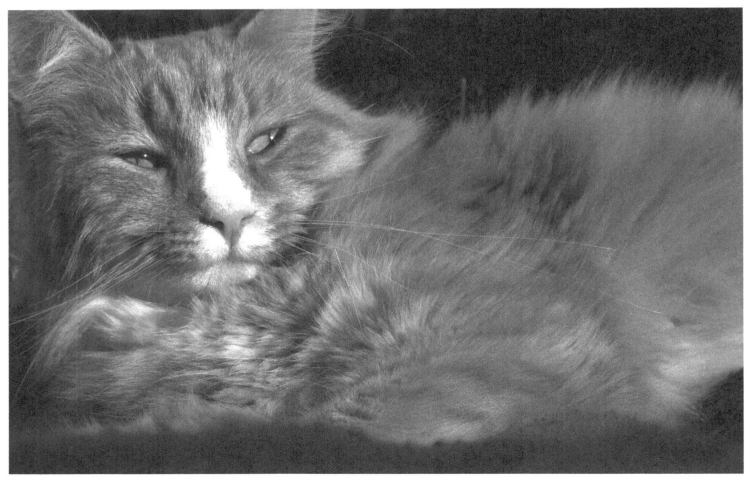

©ANGELE RICE

> " *This is what home is: not only the place you remember, but the place that remembers you, even if you have never been there before, the place that holds some essential piece of you in trust, waiting for you to return when you go out into other places in the world, as you must.* "
> —ORIAH

A place that feels like home to me: _____

The best part of my day: _____

Something that made me laugh: _____

Whom did I let "off the hook" today? _____

Someone / Something that brings me joy: _____

Where kindness touched my world today: _____

How I nourished my mind, body or spirit: _____

Number of hours I rested or slept in past 24 hours:
___ Rest   ___ Sleep

Prayer/Meditation for the day:
☼ Yes   ☼ No

I am grateful for: _____

Today I did this one little thing
    For the earth...
        for a friend or a stranger...
           for someone older or younger...
               for someone sicker...
                  in more need... _____

February 22ND

" *This is where life as I knew it changed. This is where a new feeling slowly, eventually, permeated every cell of my body, changing the way I took in the world.* "

—SHARON RAINEY

MAKING A PEARL FROM THE GRIT OF LIFE

A time or place when things changed for me: _____

The best part of my day: _____

Something that made me laugh: _____

Whom did I let "off the hook" today? _____

Someone / Something that brings me joy: _____

Where kindness touched my world today: _____

How I nourished my mind, body or spirit: _____

Number of hours I rested or slept in past 24 hours:
___Rest   ___Sleep

Prayer/Meditation for the day:
☼ Yes   ☼ No

I am grateful for: _____

Today I did this one little thing
　　For the earth...
　　　　for a friend or a stranger...
　　　　　　for someone older or younger...
　　　　　　　　for someone sicker...
　　　　　　　　　　in more need... _____

> *"Anything in life that we don't accept will simply make trouble for us until we make peace with it."*
> —SHAKTI GAWAIN

Sometime I have made peace with: _____

The best part of my day: _____

Something that made me laugh: _____

Whom did I let "off the hook" today? _____

Someone / Something that brings me joy: _____

Where kindness touched my world today: _____

How I nourished my mind, body or spirit: _____

Number of hours I rested or slept in past 24 hours:
____ Rest   ____ Sleep

Prayer/Meditation for the day:
☼ Yes   ☼ No

I am grateful for: _____

Today I did this one little thing
    For the earth...
        for a friend or a stranger...
            for someone older or younger...
                for someone sicker...
                    in more need... _____

February 24TH

"Anyone who thinks a spiritual path is easy probably hasn't been walking one."
—MARIANNE WILLIAMSON
THE AGE OF MIRACLES: EMBRACING THE NEW MIDLIFE

How I try to walk on a spiritual path: _____

The best part of my day: _____

Something that made me laugh: _____

Whom did I let "off the hook" today? _____

Someone / Something that brings me joy: _____

Where kindness touched my world today: _____

How I nourished my mind, body or spirit: _____

Number of hours I rested or slept in past 24 hours:
___ Rest   ___ Sleep

Prayer/Meditation for the day:
☼ Yes   ☼ No

I am grateful for: _____

Today I did this one little thing
    For the earth...
        for a friend or a stranger...
            for someone older or younger...
                for someone sicker...
                    in more need... _____

" Take chances, make mistakes. That's how you grow. Pain nourishes your courage. You have to fail in order to practice being brave. "
—MARY TYLER MOORE

Something I failed at that I
later realized helped me grow: _____

The best part of my day: _____

Something that made me laugh: _____

Whom did I let "off the hook" today? _____

Someone / Something that brings me joy: _____

Where kindness touched my world today: _____

How I nourished my mind, body or spirit: _____

Number of hours I rested or slept in past 24 hours:
___ Rest   ___ Sleep

Prayer/Meditation for the day:
☼ Yes   ☼ No

I am grateful for: _____

Today I did this one little thing
    For the earth...
        for a friend or a stranger...
            for someone older or younger...
                for someone sicker...
                    in more need... _____

February 26TH

> **"** *If my hands are fully occupied in holding on
> to something, I can neither give nor receive.* **"**
> —DOROTHY SOLLE

What have I allowed myself to receive: _____

The best part of my day: _____

Something that made me laugh: _____

Whom did I let "off the hook" today? _____

Someone / Something that brings me joy: _____

Where kindness touched my world today: _____

How I nourished my mind, body or spirit: _____

Number of hours I rested or slept in past 24 hours:
___ Rest   ___ Sleep

Prayer/Meditation for the day:
☼ Yes   ☼ No

I am grateful for: _____

Today I did this one little thing
    For the earth...
        for a friend or a stranger...
            for someone older or younger...
                for someone sicker...
                    in more need... _____

> *" Praise and an attitude of gratitude are unbeatable stimulators... We increase whatever we extol. "*
> —SYLVIA STITT EDWARDS

Someone I praised this week: _____

The best part of my day: _____

Something that made me laugh: _____

Whom did I let "off the hook" today? _____

Someone / Something that brings me joy: _____

Where kindness touched my world today: _____

How I nourished my mind, body or spirit: _____

Number of hours I rested or slept in past 24 hours:
____ Rest   ____ Sleep

Prayer/Meditation for the day:
☼ Yes   ☼ No

I am grateful for: _____

Today I did this one little thing
    For the earth...
        for a friend or a stranger...
            for someone older or younger...
                for someone sicker...
                    in more need... _____

February 28TH

"Joy is the feeling of grinning on the inside."
—DR. MELBA COLGROVE

Something that made me grin on the inside: _____

The best part of my day: _____

Something that made me laugh: _____

Whom did I let "off the hook" today? _____

Someone / Something that brings me joy: _____

Where kindness touched my world today: _____

How I nourished my mind, body or spirit: _____

Number of hours I rested or slept in past 24 hours:
___ Rest   ___ Sleep

Prayer/Meditation for the day:
☼ Yes   ☼ No

I am grateful for: _____

Today I did this one little thing
    For the earth...
        for a friend or a stranger...
           for someone older or younger...
               for someone sicker...
                  in more need... _____

" *Something that made me grin on the inside.* **"**
—IRVINE WELSH

What truth I have learned about my soul: _____

The best part of my day: _____

Something that made me laugh: _____

Whom did I let "off the hook" today? _____

Someone / Something that brings me joy: _____

Where kindness touched my world today: _____

How I nourished my mind, body or spirit: _____

Number of hours I rested or slept in past 24 hours:
____Rest   ____Sleep

Prayer/Meditation for the day:
☼ Yes   ☼ No

I am grateful for: _____

Today I did this one little thing
    For the earth...
        for a friend or a stranger...
           for someone older or younger...
              for someone sicker...
                in more need... _____

End of Month Review

Best part of the past ten days? _____

Number of days I laughed: _____

Goal I want to set for the next 10 days: _____

Person/people who did or
said something to help me heal: _____

Anything else I have noticed
or want to remember/record: _____

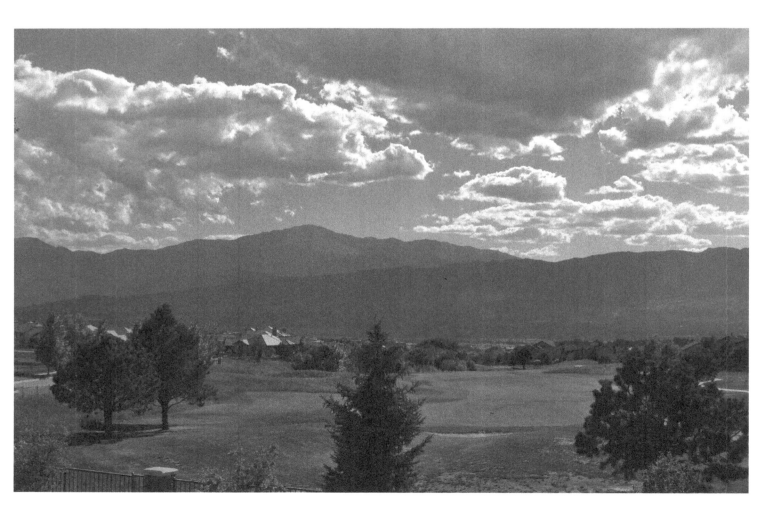

" *You have to count on living every single day in a way you believe will make you feel good about your life, so that if it were over tomorrow, you'd be content.* "
—JANE SEYMOUR

What brings contentment in my life? _____

The best part of my day: _____

Something that made me laugh: _____

Whom did I let "off the hook" today? _____

Someone / Something that brings me joy: _____

Where kindness touched my world today: _____

How I nourished my mind, body or spirit: _____

Number of hours I rested or slept in past 24 hours:
___Rest ___Sleep

Prayer/Meditation for the day:
☼ Yes ☼ No

I am grateful for: _____

Today I did this one little thing
    For the earth...
        for a friend or a stranger...
            for someone older or younger...
                for someone sicker...
                    in more need... _____

March 2ND

> "*When I let go of what I am, I become what I might be.*"
> —LAO TZU

Something I am ready to let go of: _____

The best part of my day: _____

Something that made me laugh: _____

Whom did I let "off the hook" today? _____

Someone / Something that brings me joy: _____

Where kindness touched my world today: _____

How I nourished my mind, body or spirit: _____

Number of hours I rested or slept in past 24 hours:
___ Rest   ___ Sleep

Prayer/Meditation for the day:
☼ Yes   ☼ No

I am grateful for: _____

Today I did this one little thing
    For the earth...
        for a friend or a stranger...
            for someone older or younger...
                for someone sicker...
                    in more need... _____

March 3RD

> **"** *Ultimately we know deeply that the other side of every fear is freedom.* **"**
> —MARILYN FERGUSON

I feel free when: _____

The best part of my day: _____

Something that made me laugh: _____

Whom did I let "off the hook" today? _____

Someone / Something that brings me joy: _____

Where kindness touched my world today: _____

How I nourished my mind, body or spirit: _____

Number of hours I rested or slept in past 24 hours:
___ Rest ___ Sleep

Prayer/Meditation for the day:
☼ Yes ☼ No

I am grateful for: _____

Today I did this one little thing
   For the earth...
      for a friend or a stranger...
         for someone older or younger...
           for someone sicker...
              in more need... _____

March 4ᵀᴴ

" It helps, I think, to consider ourselves on a very long journey: the main thing is to keep to the faith, to endure, to help each other when we stumble or tire, to weep and press on. "
—MARY CAROLINE RICHARDS

How I showed my faith today: _____

The best part of my day: _____

Something that made me laugh: _____

Whom did I let "off the hook" today? _____

Someone / Something that brings me joy: _____

Where kindness touched my world today: _____

How I nourished my mind, body or spirit: _____

Number of hours I rested or slept in past 24 hours:
___ Rest   ___ Sleep

Prayer/Meditation for the day:
☼ Yes   ☼ No

I am grateful for: _____

Today I did this one little thing
    For the earth...
        for a friend or a stranger...
            for someone older or younger...
                for someone sicker...
                    in more need... _____

> " *Most of all, I remember her laughing. It filled my ears. Her smile, her sparkling eyes, and her infectious laughter, along with the vistas, were limitless and unending and powerful.* "
>
> —SHARON RAINEY
> *MAKING A PEARL FROM THE GRIT OF LIFE*

Someone's laugh you love to hear: _____

The best part of my day: _____

Something that made me laugh: _____

Whom did I let "off the hook" today? _____

Someone / Something that brings me joy: _____

Where kindness touched my world today: _____

How I nourished my mind, body or spirit: _____

Number of hours I rested or slept in past 24 hours:
___ Rest ___ Sleep

Prayer/Meditation for the day:
☼ Yes ☼ No

I am grateful for: _____

Today I did this one little thing
For the earth...
for a friend or a stranger...
for someone older or younger...
for someone sicker...
in more need... _____

March 6ᵀᴴ

" If anything matters then everything matters. Because you are important, everything you do is important. Every time you forgive, the universe changes; every time you reach out and touch a heart or a life, the world changes; with every kindness and service, seen or unseen, God's purposes are accomplished and nothing will ever be the same again."

—WM PAUL YOUNG
THE SHACK

Three things I touched today: _____

The best part of my day: _____

Something that made me laugh: _____

Whom did I let "off the hook" today? _____

Someone / Something that brings me joy: _____

Where kindness touched my world today: _____

How I nourished my mind, body or spirit: _____

Number of hours I rested or slept in past 24 hours:
____ Rest   ____ Sleep

Prayer/Meditation for the day:
☼ Yes   ☼ No

I am grateful for: _____

Today I did this one little thing
    For the earth...
        for a friend or a stranger...
           for someone older or younger...
               for someone sicker...
                  in more need... _____

> **"***It's ok to do less than is humanly possible.***"**
> —ANONYMOUS

I need: _____

The best part of my day: _____

Something that made me laugh: _____

Whom did I let "off the hook" today? _____

Someone / Something that brings me joy: _____

Where kindness touched my world today: _____

How I nourished my mind, body or spirit: _____

Number of hours I rested or slept in past 24 hours:
___Rest   ___Sleep

Prayer/Meditation for the day:
☼ Yes   ☼ No

I am grateful for: _____

Today I did this one little thing
　　For the earth...
　　　　for a friend or a stranger...
　　　　　　for someone older or younger...
　　　　　　　　for someone sicker...
　　　　　　　　　　in more need... _____

March 8TH

" That is happiness: to be dissolved into something completely great. "
—WILLA CATHER

What brought me happiness today: _____

The best part of my day: _____

Something that made me laugh: _____

Whom did I let "off the hook" today? _____

Someone / Something that brings me joy: _____

Where kindness touched my world today: _____

How I nourished my mind, body or spirit: _____

Number of hours I rested or slept in past 24 hours:
____Rest   ____Sleep

Prayer/Meditation for the day:
☼ Yes   ☼ No

I am grateful for: _____

Today I did this one little thing
    For the earth...
        for a friend or a stranger...
            for someone older or younger...
                for someone sicker...
                    in more need... _____

> **"** *Children, like animals, use all their senses to discover the world.*
> *Then artists come along and discover it the same way all over again.* **"**
> —EUDORA WELTY

The last time I petted an animal: _____

The best part of my day: _____

Something that made me laugh: _____

Whom did I let "off the hook" today? _____

Someone / Something that brings me joy: _____

Where kindness touched my world today: _____

How I nourished my mind, body or spirit: _____

Number of hours I rested or slept in past 24 hours:
____Rest   ____Sleep

Prayer/Meditation for the day:
☼ Yes   ☼ No

I am grateful for: _____

Today I did this one little thing
   For the earth...
      for a friend or a stranger...
         for someone older or younger...
            for someone sicker...
               in more need... _____

March 10TH

"It takes courage to lead a life. Any life."
—ERICA JONG

How/When I demonstrated courage: _____

The best part of my day: _____

Something that made me laugh: _____

Whom did I let "off the hook" today? _____

Someone / Something that brings me joy: _____

Where kindness touched my world today: _____

How I nourished my mind, body or spirit: _____

Number of hours I rested or slept in past 24 hours:
____Rest   ____Sleep

Prayer/Meditation for the day:
☼ Yes   ☼ No

I am grateful for: _____

Today I did this one little thing
    For the earth...
        for a friend or a stranger...
            for someone older or younger...
                for someone sicker...
                    in more need... _____

Early Month Review

Best part of the past ten days? _____

Number of days I laughed: _____

Goal I want to set for the next 10 days: _____

Person/people who did or
said something to help me heal: _____

Anything else I have noticed
or want to remember/record: _____

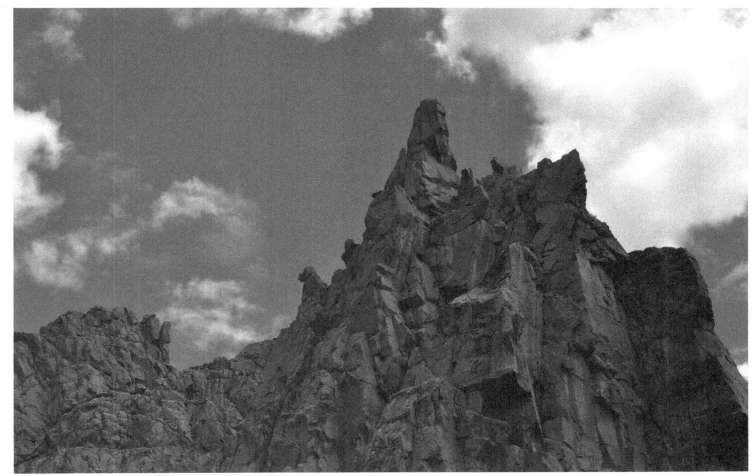

©STEPHEN RAINEY

March 11TH

"*When you act out of fear, your fears come true.*"
—DAVID BAYLES, TED ORLAND
ART & FEAR: OBSERVATIONS ON THE PERILS (AND REWARDS) OF ARTMAKING

What am I acting out of today? _____

The best part of my day: _____

Something that made me laugh: _____

Whom did I let "off the hook" today? _____

Someone / Something that brings me joy: _____

Where kindness touched my world today: _____

How I nourished my mind, body or spirit: _____

Number of hours I rested or slept in past 24 hours:
___ Rest ___ Sleep

Prayer/Meditation for the day:
☼ Yes ☼ No

I am grateful for: _____

Today I did this one little thing
    For the earth...
        for a friend or a stranger...
           for someone older or younger...
             for someone sicker...
                in more need... _____

March 12TH

> "*Kindness is the ability to love people more than they deserve.*"
> —ANONYMOUS

Someone I love more than they deserve: _____

The best part of my day: _____

Something that made me laugh: _____

Whom did I let "off the hook" today? _____

Someone / Something that brings me joy: _____

Where kindness touched my world today: _____

How I nourished my mind, body or spirit: _____

Number of hours I rested or slept in past 24 hours:
___ Rest   ___ Sleep

Prayer/Meditation for the day:
☼ Yes   ☼ No

I am grateful for: _____

Today I did this one little thing
    For the earth...
        for a friend or a stranger...
            for someone older or younger...
                for someone sicker...
                    in more need... _____

March 13TH

"Once I decide to do something, I can't have people telling me I can't. If there's a roadblock, you jump over it, walk around it, crawl under it."
—KITTY KELLEY

A roadblock I circumnavigated: _____

The best part of my day: _____

Something that made me laugh: _____

Whom did I let "off the hook" today? _____

Someone / Something that brings me joy: _____

Where kindness touched my world today: _____

How I nourished my mind, body or spirit: _____

Number of hours I rested or slept in past 24 hours:
___ Rest   ___ Sleep

Prayer/Meditation for the day:
☼ Yes   ☼ No

I am grateful for: _____

Today I did this one little thing
    For the earth...
        for a friend or a stranger...
           for someone older or younger...
               for someone sicker...
                  in more need... _____

> **"** *Though we travel the world over to find the
> beautiful, we must carry it with us or we find it not.* **"**
> —RALPH WALDO EMERSON

Something that calmed me today: _____

The best part of my day: _____

Something that made me laugh: _____

Whom did I let "off the hook" today? _____

Someone / Something that brings me joy: _____

Where kindness touched my world today: _____

How I nourished my mind, body or spirit: _____

Number of hours I rested or slept in past 24 hours:
___ Rest   ___ Sleep

Prayer/Meditation for the day:
☼ Yes   ☼ No

I am grateful for: _____

Today I did this one little thing
    For the earth...
        for a friend or a stranger...
            for someone older or younger...
                for someone sicker...
                    in more need... _____

March 15TH

"A year or so ago I went through all the people in my life and asked myself: does this person inspire me, genuinely love me and support me unconditionally? I wanted nothing but positive influences in my life."
—MENA SUVARI

Is there anyone I need to let go of in my life? _____

The best part of my day: _____

Something that made me laugh: _____

Whom did I let "off the hook" today? _____

Someone / Something that brings me joy: _____

Where kindness touched my world today: _____

How I nourished my mind, body or spirit: _____

Number of hours I rested or slept in past 24 hours:
___ Rest ___ Sleep

Prayer/Meditation for the day:
☀ Yes ☀ No

I am grateful for: _____

Today I did this one little thing
    For the earth...
        for a friend or a stranger...
            for someone older or younger...
                for someone sicker...
                    in more need... _____

> " *It takes more courage to reveal insecurities than to hide them, more strength to relate to people than to dominate them, more 'manhood' to abide by thought-out principles rather than blind reflex. Toughness is in the soul and spirit, not in muscles and an immature mind.* "
>
> —ALEX KARRAS

Something that nourished my soul: _____

The best part of my day: _____

Something that made me laugh: _____

Whom did I let "off the hook" today? _____

Someone / Something that brings me joy: _____

Where kindness touched my world today: _____

How I nourished my mind, body or spirit: _____

Number of hours I rested or slept in past 24 hours:
___ Rest ___ Sleep

Prayer/Meditation for the day:
☼ Yes ☼ No

I am grateful for: _____

Today I did this one little thing
    For the earth...
        for a friend or a stranger...
            for someone older or younger...
                for someone sicker...
                    in more need... _____

March 17TH

" *To thine own self be true.* "
—WILLIAM SHAKESPEARE

How am I staying true to myself today? _____

The best part of my day: _____

Something that made me laugh: _____

Whom did I let "off the hook" today? _____

Someone / Something that brings me joy: _____

Where kindness touched my world today: _____

How I nourished my mind, body or spirit: _____

Number of hours I rested or slept in past 24 hours:
_____ Rest   _____ Sleep

Prayer/Meditation for the day:
☀ Yes   ☀ No

I am grateful for: _____

Today I did this one little thing
    For the earth...
        for a friend or a stranger...
           for someone older or younger...
             for someone sicker...
                in more need... _____

> **"***Sometimes life's miracles are not just handed to us, not just simply revealed when we are ready to see, but instead they require work.***"**
>
> —JEANNE SELANDER MILLER
> *A BREATH AWAY*

What work do I need to do today? _____

The best part of my day: _____

Something that made me laugh: _____

Whom did I let "off the hook" today? _____

Someone / Something that brings me joy: _____

Where kindness touched my world today: _____

How I nourished my mind, body or spirit: _____

Number of hours I rested or slept in past 24 hours:
___ Rest ___ Sleep

Prayer/Meditation for the day:
☼ Yes ☼ No

I am grateful for: _____

Today I did this one little thing
    For the earth...
        for a friend or a stranger...
           for someone older or younger...
              for someone sicker...
                in more need... _____

March 19TH

"Leap and the net will appear."
—ZEN SAYING

Am I am listening to my intuition? _____

The best part of my day: _____

Something that made me laugh: _____

Whom did I let "off the hook" today? _____

Someone / Something that brings me joy: _____

Where kindness touched my world today: _____

How I nourished my mind, body or spirit: _____

Number of hours I rested or slept in past 24 hours:
___ Rest   ___ Sleep

Prayer/Meditation for the day:
☼ Yes   ☼ No

I am grateful for: _____

Today I did this one little thing
    For the earth...
        for a friend or a stranger...
           for someone older or younger...
             for someone sicker...
                in more need... _____

> " *Hang onto hope, until you don't need it anymore. You*
> *will know this when love has come to take its place.* "
> —KEVIN DRUMMOND

I feel hopeful about: _____

The best part of my day: _____

Something that made me laugh: _____

Whom did I let "off the hook" today? _____

Someone / Something that brings me joy: _____

Where kindness touched my world today: _____

How I nourished my mind, body or spirit: _____

Number of hours I rested or slept in past 24 hours:

___ Rest   ___ Sleep

Prayer/Meditation for the day:

☼ Yes   ☼ No

I am grateful for: _____

Today I did this one little thing

    For the earth...

        for a friend or a stranger...

            for someone older or younger...

                for someone sicker...

                    in more need... _____

Mid Month
Review

Best part of the past ten days? _____

Number of days I laughed: _____

Goal I want to set for the next 10 days: _____

Person/people who did or
said something to help me heal: _____

Anything else I have noticed
or want to remember/record: _____

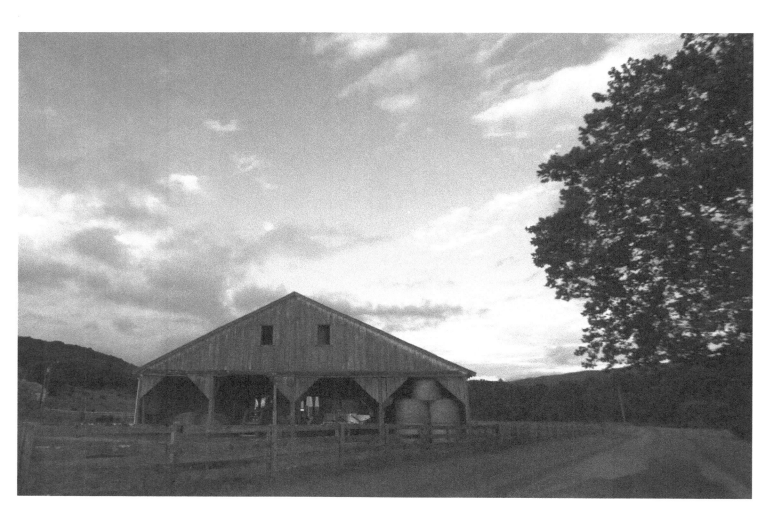

"*Life is like a prism. What you see depends on how you turn the glass.*"
—JONATHAN KELLERMAN

Today I see: _____

The best part of my day: _____

Something that made me laugh: _____

Whom did I let "off the hook" today? _____

Someone / Something that brings me joy: _____

Where kindness touched my world today: _____

How I nourished my mind, body or spirit: _____

Number of hours I rested or slept in past 24 hours:
___ Rest   ___ Sleep

Prayer/Meditation for the day:
☼ Yes   ☼ No

I am grateful for: _____

Today I did this one little thing
    For the earth...
        for a friend or a stranger...
           for someone older or younger...
               for someone sicker...
                  in more need... _____

March 22ND

"Every time you put something in your mouth,
you either feed your body or feed your disease."
—SHARON RAINEY

What did I feed today? _____

The best part of my day: _____

Something that made me laugh: _____

Whom did I let "off the hook" today? _____

Someone / Something that brings me joy: _____

Where kindness touched my world today: _____

How I nourished my mind, body or spirit: _____

Number of hours I rested or slept in past 24 hours:
___ Rest ___ Sleep

Prayer/Meditation for the day:
☼ Yes ☼ No

I am grateful for: _____

Today I did this one little thing
    For the earth...
        for a friend or a stranger...
            for someone older or younger...
                for someone sicker...
                    in more need... _____

> **"** *Two roads diverged in a wood, and I, I took the one less traveled by, And that has made all the difference.* **"**
> —ROBERT FROST

When I took a chance I wouldn't normally take: _____

The best part of my day: _____

Something that made me laugh: _____

Whom did I let "off the hook" today? _____

Someone / Something that brings me joy: _____

Where kindness touched my world today: _____

How I nourished my mind, body or spirit: _____

Number of hours I rested or slept in past 24 hours:
___Rest   ___Sleep

Prayer/Meditation for the day:
☼ Yes   ☼ No

I am grateful for: _____

Today I did this one little thing
    For the earth...
        for a friend or a stranger...
            for someone older or younger...
                for someone sicker...
                    in more need... _____

March 24TH

> *"You can't do anything about the length of your life,*
> *but you can do something about its width and depth."*
> —H.L. MENCKEN

What or who gave me energy today: _____

The best part of my day: _____

Something that made me laugh: _____

Whom did I let "off the hook" today? _____

Someone / Something that brings me joy: _____

Where kindness touched my world today: _____

How I nourished my mind, body or spirit: _____

Number of hours I rested or slept in past 24 hours:
___ Rest ___ Sleep

Prayer/Meditation for the day:
☼ Yes ☼ No

I am grateful for: _____

Today I did this one little thing
    For the earth...
        for a friend or a stranger...
           for someone older or younger...
              for someone sicker...
                in more need... _____

"*Art is the triumph over chaos.*"
—JOHN CHEEVER

Favorite color and how it makes me feel: _____

The best part of my day: _____

Something that made me laugh: _____

Whom did I let "off the hook" today? _____

Someone / Something that brings me joy: _____

Where kindness touched my world today: _____

How I nourished my mind, body or spirit: _____

Number of hours I rested or slept in past 24 hours:
____ Rest   ____ Sleep

Prayer/Meditation for the day:
☼ Yes   ☼ No

I am grateful for: _____

Today I did this one little thing
    For the earth...
        for a friend or a stranger...
            for someone older or younger...
                for someone sicker...
                    in more need... _____

March 26TH

"If you have built castles in the air, your work need not be lost;
that is where they should be. Now put foundations under them."
—HENRY DAVID THOREAU

I honor myself for _____ .

The best part of my day: _____

Something that made me laugh: _____

Whom did I let "off the hook" today? _____

Someone / Something that brings me joy: _____

Where kindness touched my world today: _____

How I nourished my mind, body or spirit: _____

Number of hours I rested or slept in past 24 hours:
___ Rest   ___ Sleep

Prayer/Meditation for the day:
☼ Yes   ☼ No

I am grateful for: _____

Today I did this one little thing
    For the earth...
        for a friend or a stranger...
            for someone older or younger...
                for someone sicker...
                    in more need... _____

" *Out of clutter, find simplicity. From discord, find harmony. In the middle of difficulty lies opportunity.* **"**
—ALBERT EINSTEIN

An opportunity or something simple I saw: _____

The best part of my day: _____

Something that made me laugh: _____

Whom did I let "off the hook" today? _____

Someone / Something that brings me joy: _____

Where kindness touched my world today: _____

How I nourished my mind, body or spirit: _____

Number of hours I rested or slept in past 24 hours:
___ Rest ___ Sleep

Prayer/Meditation for the day:
☼ Yes   ☼ No

I am grateful for: _____

Today I did this one little thing
　　For the earth...
　　　　for a friend or a stranger...
　　　　　　for someone older or younger...
　　　　　　　　for someone sicker...
　　　　　　　　　　in more need... _____

March 28TH

"*Scared is what you're feeling. Brave is what you're doing.*"
—EMMA DONOGHUE

What I did recently that was brave despite my fear: _____

The best part of my day: _____

Something that made me laugh: _____

Whom did I let "off the hook" today? _____

Someone / Something that brings me joy: _____

Where kindness touched my world today: _____

How I nourished my mind, body or spirit: _____

Number of hours I rested or slept in past 24 hours:
____ Rest   ____ Sleep

Prayer/Meditation for the day:
☼ Yes   ☼ No

I am grateful for: _____

Today I did this one little thing
     For the earth...
          for a friend or a stranger...
               for someone older or younger...
                    for someone sicker...
                         in more need... _____

> **"** *There is an odd synchronicity in the way parallel lives veer to touch one another, change direction, and then come close again and again until they connect and hold for whatever it was that fate intended to happen.* **"**
> —ANN RULE

Where do I see synchronicity today? _____

The best part of my day: _____

Something that made me laugh: _____

Whom did I let "off the hook" today? _____

Someone / Something that brings me joy: _____

Where kindness touched my world today: _____

How I nourished my mind, body or spirit: _____

Number of hours I rested or slept in past 24 hours:
___ Rest   ___ Sleep

Prayer/Meditation for the day:
☼ Yes   ☼ No

I am grateful for: _____

Today I did this one little thing
    For the earth...
        for a friend or a stranger...
            for someone older or younger...
                for someone sicker...
                    in more need... _____

March 30TH

"May you trust that you are exactly where you are meant to be. May you not forget the infinite possibilities that are born of faith in yourself and others. May you use the gifts that you have received, and pass on the love that has been given to you. May you be content with yourself just the way you are. Let this knowledge settle into your bones, and allow your soul the freedom to sing, dance, praise and love. It is there for each and every one of us."

—SAINT TERESE OF LISEAUX

What can I accept about myself today that
I have previously had difficulty accepting? _____

The best part of my day: _____

Something that made me laugh: _____

Whom did I let "off the hook" today? _____

Someone / Something that brings me joy: _____

Where kindness touched my world today: _____

How I nourished my mind, body or spirit: _____

Number of hours I rested or slept in past 24 hours:
___ Rest   ___ Sleep

Prayer/Meditation for the day:
☼ Yes   ☼ No

I am grateful for: _____

Today I did this one little thing
    For the earth...
        for a friend or a stranger...
            for someone older or younger...
                for someone sicker...
                    in more need... _____

March 31ST

"Earth has no sorrow that heaven cannot heal."
—THOMAS MOORE

What needs healing in my soul? _____

The best part of my day: _____

Something that made me laugh: _____

Whom did I let "off the hook" today? _____

Someone / Something that brings me joy: _____

Where kindness touched my world today: _____

How I nourished my mind, body or spirit: _____

Number of hours I rested or slept in past 24 hours:
___ Rest ___ Sleep

Prayer/Meditation for the day:
☼ Yes ☼ No

I am grateful for: _____

Today I did this one little thing
    For the earth...
        for a friend or a stranger...
            for someone older or younger...
                for someone sicker...
                    in more need... _____

End of Month Review

Best part of the past ten days? _____

Number of days I laughed: _____

Goal I want to set for the next 10 days: _____

Person/people who did or
said something to help me heal: _____

Anything else I have noticed
or want to remember/record: _____

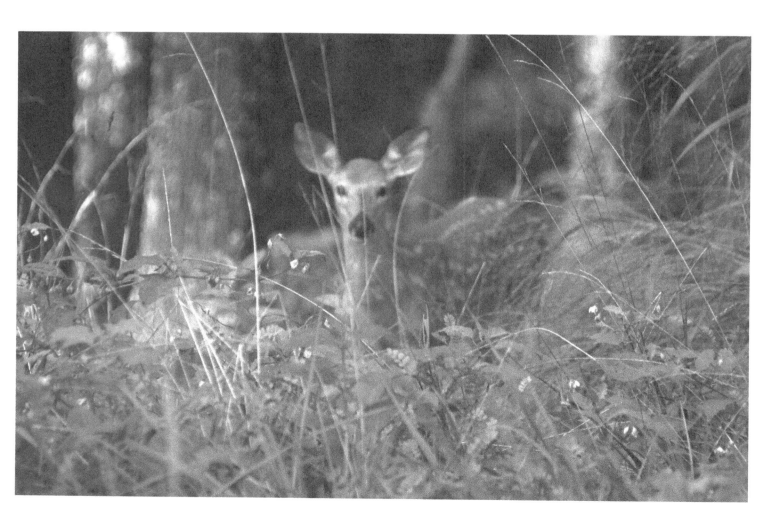

" It was beyond her and she knew it. She knelt down in its intensity.
Gratitude filled her, tears cleansed her and energy flowed thru her.. "
—TERRI ST. CLOUD
BONESIGHARTS.COM

I am grateful for: _____

The best part of my day: _____

Something that made me laugh: _____

Whom did I let "off the hook" today? _____

Someone / Something that brings me joy: _____

Where kindness touched my world today: _____

How I nourished my mind, body or spirit: _____

Number of hours I rested or slept in past 24 hours:
___ Rest   ___ Sleep

Prayer/Meditation for the day:
☼ Yes   ☼ No

I am grateful for: _____

Today I did this one little thing
    For the earth...
        for a friend or a stranger...
           for someone older or younger...
               for someone sicker...
                  in more need... _____

April 2ND

"It is not the length of your experience that qualifies you; it's the depth of it!"
—CATHY HOLLOWAY HILL

A profound experience I had: _____

The best part of my day: _____

Something that made me laugh: _____

Whom did I let "off the hook" today? _____

Someone / Something that brings me joy: _____

Where kindness touched my world today: _____

How I nourished my mind, body or spirit: _____

Number of hours I rested or slept in past 24 hours:
___ Rest   ___ Sleep

Prayer/Meditation for the day:
☼ Yes   ☼ No

I am grateful for: _____

Today I did this one little thing
    For the earth...
        for a friend or a stranger...
           for someone older or younger...
               for someone sicker...
                  in more need... _____

> *" Fall down seven times; get up eight times. "*
> —JAPANESE PROVERB

Am I willing to get back up? _____

The best part of my day: _____

Something that made me laugh: _____

Whom did I let "off the hook" today? _____

Someone / Something that brings me joy: _____

Where kindness touched my world today: _____

How I nourished my mind, body or spirit: _____

Number of hours I rested or slept in past 24 hours:
___ Rest ___ Sleep

Prayer/Meditation for the day:
☼ Yes ☼ No

I am grateful for: _____

Today I did this one little thing
 For the earth...
  for a friend or a stranger...
   for someone older or younger...
    for someone sicker...
     in more need... _____

April 4TH

"Be a duck; let the negativity roll right off your back."
—JEFF RAINEY

I accept the fact that: _____

The best part of my day: _____

Something that made me laugh: _____

Whom did I let "off the hook" today? _____

Someone / Something that brings me joy: _____

Where kindness touched my world today: _____

How I nourished my mind, body or spirit: _____

Number of hours I rested or slept in past 24 hours:
___ Rest   ___ Sleep

Prayer/Meditation for the day:
☼ Yes   ☼ No

I am grateful for: _____

Today I did this one little thing
    For the earth...
        for a friend or a stranger...
            for someone older or younger...
                for someone sicker...
                    in more need... _____

April 5TH

"I believe there are many sources of healing energy that cannot be prescribed, surgically implanted, or analyzed by blood tests. We need to learn how to access that energy source to heal ourselves and help others. Each of us has the ability to do that. Tapping into that infinite energy source takes practice, dedication, and refinement of skills. Based on my own personal experience, there is much to learn from seeking out gifted individuals and alternative healers — especially when we act proactively and in a preventive mode before we get seriously ill."
—DR. NEIL SPECTOR

What healing energy will I tap into today? _____

The best part of my day: _____

Something that made me laugh: _____

Whom did I let "off the hook" today? _____

Someone / Something that brings me joy: _____

Where kindness touched my world today: _____

How I nourished my mind, body or spirit: _____

Number of hours I rested or slept in past 24 hours:
___ Rest   ___ Sleep

Prayer/Meditation for the day:
☼ Yes   ☼ No

I am grateful for: _____

Today I did this one little thing
   For the earth...
      for a friend or a stranger...
         for someone older or younger...
            for someone sicker...
               in more need... _____

April 6TH

"It is during our darkest moments that we must focus to see the light."
—ARISTOTLE ONASSIS

What light can I see today? _____

The best part of my day: _____

Something that made me laugh: _____

Whom did I let "off the hook" today? _____

Someone / Something that brings me joy: _____

Where kindness touched my world today: _____

How I nourished my mind, body or spirit: _____

Number of hours I rested or slept in past 24 hours:
___ Rest ___ Sleep

Prayer/Meditation for the day:
☼ Yes ☼ No

I am grateful for: _____

Today I did this one little thing
  For the earth...
    for a friend or a stranger...
      for someone older or younger...
        for someone sicker...
          in more need... _____

"*Everything I think, everything I do, is based in love or in fear. It's my choice.*"
—SHARON RAINEY

Am I living today in fear or love? _____

The best part of my day: _____

Something that made me laugh: _____

Whom did I let "off the hook" today? _____

Someone / Something that brings me joy: _____

Where kindness touched my world today: _____

How I nourished my mind, body or spirit: _____

Number of hours I rested or slept in past 24 hours:
___Rest   ___Sleep

Prayer/Meditation for the day:
☼ Yes   ☼ No

I am grateful for: _____

Today I did this one little thing
    For the earth...
        for a friend or a stranger...
            for someone older or younger...
                for someone sicker...
                    in more need... _____

April 8TH

"Look at the choices you have, as opposed to the choices that have been taken away from you. Because in those choices, there are whole worlds of strength and new ways to look at things."

—MICHAEL J. FOX

What choices do I have today? _____

The best part of my day: _____

Something that made me laugh: _____

Whom did I let "off the hook" today? _____

Someone / Something that brings me joy: _____

Where kindness touched my world today: _____

How I nourished my mind, body or spirit: _____

Number of hours I rested or slept in past 24 hours:
___ Rest   ___ Sleep

Prayer/Meditation for the day:
☼ Yes   ☼ No

I am grateful for: _____

Today I did this one little thing
    For the earth...
        for a friend or a stranger...
           for someone older or younger...
             for someone sicker...
               in more need... _____

> " *All you can work on today is directly in front of you.*
> *Your job is to develop an imagination of the possible.* "
> —DAVID BAYLES, TED ORLAND
> *ART & FEAR: OBSERVATIONS ON THE PERILS (AND REWARDS) OF ARTMAKING*

What can I imagine doing
today that will help me heal? _____

The best part of my day: _____

Something that made me laugh: _____

Whom did I let "off the hook" today? _____

Someone / Something that brings me joy: _____

Where kindness touched my world today: _____

How I nourished my mind, body or spirit: _____

Number of hours I rested or slept in past 24 hours:
___ Rest   ___ Sleep

Prayer/Meditation for the day:
☼ Yes   ☼ No

I am grateful for: _____

Today I did this one little thing
    For the earth...
        for a friend or a stranger...
            for someone older or younger...
                for someone sicker...
                    in more need... _____

April 10TH

" *True knowledge comes only through suffering.* "
—ELIZABETH BARRETT BROWNING

Three things I've learned while healing: _____

The best part of my day: _____

Something that made me laugh: _____

Whom did I let "off the hook" today? _____

Someone / Something that brings me joy: _____

Where kindness touched my world today: _____

How I nourished my mind, body or spirit: _____

Number of hours I rested or slept in past 24 hours:
___ Rest   ___ Sleep

Prayer/Meditation for the day:
☼ Yes   ☼ No

I am grateful for: _____

Today I did this one little thing
   For the earth...
      for a friend or a stranger...
         for someone older or younger...
           for someone sicker...
              in more need... _____

Early Month Review

Best part of the past ten days? _____

Number of days I laughed: _____

Goal I want to set for the next 10 days: _____

Person/people who did or
said something to help me heal: _____

Anything else I have noticed
or want to remember/record: _____

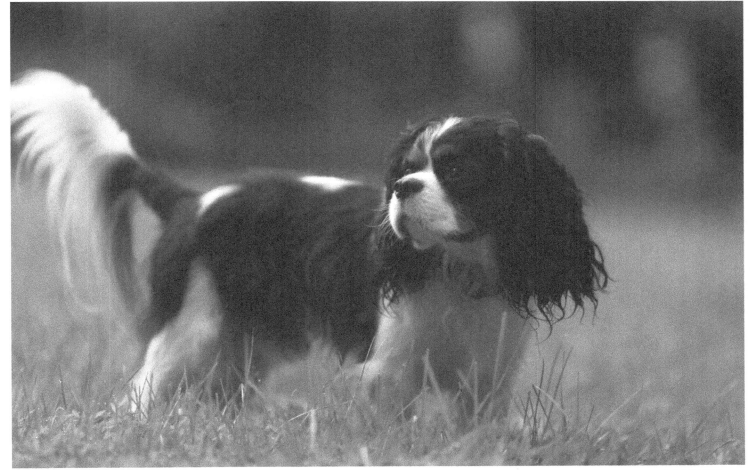

©JOE KELLY

April 11TH

> *"As for the many people who ask for the formula I used to get to where I am: there is not one clear answer I am ever able to give other than to become the very best version of yourself during your journey, find a doctor you trust and surround yourself with people who love and support you."*
>
> —ALYSSA KNAPP

Who am I surrounding myself with? _____

The best part of my day: _____

Something that made me laugh: _____

Whom did I let "off the hook" today? _____

Someone / Something that brings me joy: _____

Where kindness touched my world today: _____

How I nourished my mind, body or spirit: _____

Number of hours I rested or slept in past 24 hours:
___ Rest   ___ Sleep

Prayer/Meditation for the day:
☼ Yes   ☼ No

I am grateful for: _____

Today I did this one little thing
    For the earth...
        for a friend or a stranger...
            for someone older or younger...
                for someone sicker...
                    in more need... _____

> " *Hate begets hate; violence begets violence; toughness begets a greater toughness. We must meet the forces of hate with the power of love.* "
> —MARTIN LUTHER KING, JR.

Someone I dealt with in a kind,
gentle way or someone I protected: _____

The best part of my day: _____

Something that made me laugh: _____

Whom did I let "off the hook" today? _____

Someone / Something that brings me joy: _____

Where kindness touched my world today: _____

How I nourished my mind, body or spirit: _____

Number of hours I rested or slept in past 24 hours:
___ Rest   ___ Sleep

Prayer/Meditation for the day:
☼ Yes   ☼ No

I am grateful for: _____

Today I did this one little thing
   For the earth...
      for a friend or a stranger...
         for someone older or younger...
           for someone sicker...
             in more need... _____

April 13TH

> " *The garden is growth and change, and that means loss as*
> *well as constant new treasures to make up for a few disasters.* "
> —MARY SARTON

What new treasure have I reacently uncovered? _____

The best part of my day: _____

Something that made me laugh: _____

Whom did I let "off the hook" today? _____

Someone / Something that brings me joy: _____

Where kindness touched my world today: _____

How I nourished my mind, body or spirit: _____

Number of hours I rested or slept in past 24 hours:
___ Rest   ___ Sleep

Prayer/Meditation for the day:
☼ Yes   ☼ No

I am grateful for: _____

Today I did this one little thing
    For the earth...
        for a friend or a stranger...
           for someone older or younger...
               for someone sicker...
                  in more need... _____

" *Don't judge each day by the harvest you reap, but by the seeds you plant.* "
—ROBERT LOUIS STEVENSON

I started: _____

The best part of my day: _____

Something that made me laugh: _____

Whom did I let "off the hook" today? _____

Someone / Something that brings me joy: _____

Where kindness touched my world today: _____

How I nourished my mind, body or spirit: _____

Number of hours I rested or slept in past 24 hours:
___ Rest   ___ Sleep

Prayer/Meditation for the day:
☼ Yes   ☼ No

I am grateful for: _____

Today I did this one little thing
  For the earth...
    for a friend or a stranger...
      for someone older or younger...
        for someone sicker...
          in more need... _____

April 15TH

" Pain is your best friend. It is infinitely more honest with you than pleasure. Despite what you might think, the painful experiences you have had benefit you far more than the pleasurable ones, even though most of us spend our lives trying to duck and hide from them. But when you can center yourself and be open to look pain dead in the eye, then you have transcended the limits of your ego and this humanity. It is then that you enter into the possibility of becoming a great being. "

—SWAMI CHETANANANDA

DYNAMIC STILLNESS, RUDRA PUBLICATION, 2001

Do I believe I am becoming a great being? _____

The best part of my day: _____

Something that made me laugh: _____

Whom did I let "off the hook" today? _____

Someone / Something that brings me joy: _____

Where kindness touched my world today: _____

How I nourished my mind, body or spirit: _____

Number of hours I rested or slept in past 24 hours:
____ Rest   ____ Sleep

Prayer/Meditation for the day:
☼ Yes   ☼ No

I am grateful for: _____

Today I did this one little thing
　　For the earth...
　　　　for a friend or a stranger...
　　　　　　for someone older or younger...
　　　　　　　　for someone sicker...
　　　　　　　　　　in more need... _____

" *Now I look for ways to alleviate some of the fatigue, because even small reductions in that symptom can have a major impact on a patient's sense of hope.* "
—JEROME GROOPMAN

What or who gave me energy today: _____

The best part of my day: _____

Something that made me laugh: _____

Whom did I let "off the hook" today? _____

Someone / Something that brings me joy: _____

Where kindness touched my world today: _____

How I nourished my mind, body or spirit: _____

Number of hours I rested or slept in past 24 hours:
___ Rest   ___ Sleep

Prayer/Meditation for the day:
☼ Yes   ☼ No

I am grateful for: _____

Today I did this one little thing
    For the earth...
        for a friend or a stranger...
            for someone older or younger...
                for someone sicker...
                    in more need... _____

April 17ᵀᴴ

> " *If you don't go after what you want, you'll never have it. If you don't ask, the answer is always no. If you don't step forward, you're always in the same place.* "
> —NORA ROBERTS

How will I step forward today? _____

The best part of my day: _____

Something that made me laugh: _____

Whom did I let "off the hook" today? _____

Someone / Something that brings me joy: _____

Where kindness touched my world today: _____

How I nourished my mind, body or spirit: _____

Number of hours I rested or slept in past 24 hours:
___ Rest   ___ Sleep

Prayer/Meditation for the day:
☼ Yes   ☼ No

I am grateful for: _____

Today I did this one little thing
    For the earth...
        for a friend or a stranger...
           for someone older or younger...
                for someone sicker...
                    in more need... _____

"*When patterns are broken, new worlds emerge.*"
—TULI KUPFERBERG

What I can see emerging: _____

The best part of my day: _____

Something that made me laugh: _____

Whom did I let "off the hook" today? _____

Someone / Something that brings me joy: _____

Where kindness touched my world today: _____

How I nourished my mind, body or spirit: _____

Number of hours I rested or slept in past 24 hours:
___ Rest ___ Sleep

Prayer/Meditation for the day:
☼ Yes ☼ No

I am grateful for: _____

Today I did this one little thing
    For the earth...
        for a friend or a stranger...
           for someone older or younger...
              for someone sicker...
                in more need... _____

April 19TH

"I've learned from experience that the greater part of our happiness or misery depends on our dispositions and not on our circumstances."
—MARTHA WASHINGTON

I am glad that: _____

The best part of my day: _____

Something that made me laugh: _____

Whom did I let "off the hook" today? _____

Someone / Something that brings me joy: _____

Where kindness touched my world today: _____

How I nourished my mind, body or spirit: _____

Number of hours I rested or slept in past 24 hours:
____ Rest   ____ Sleep

Prayer/Meditation for the day:
☼ Yes   ☼ No

I am grateful for: _____

Today I did this one little thing
    For the earth...
        for a friend or a stranger...
           for someone older or younger...
               for someone sicker...
                   in more need... _____

"Enthusiasm is excitement with inspiration, motivation, and a pinch of creativity."
—BO BENNETT
YEAR TO SUCCESS: WHEN IT COMES TO SUCCESS, THERE ARE NO SHORTCUTS

Someone who inspires me: _____

The best part of my day: _____

Something that made me laugh: _____

Whom did I let "off the hook" today? _____

Someone / Something that brings me joy: _____

Where kindness touched my world today: _____

How I nourished my mind, body or spirit: _____

Number of hours I rested or slept in past 24 hours:
___ Rest   ___ Sleep

Prayer/Meditation for the day:
☼ Yes   ☼ No

I am grateful for: _____

Today I did this one little thing
        For the earth...
                for a friend or a stranger...
                        for someone older or younger...
                                for someone sicker...
                                        in more need... _____

Mid Month
Review

Best part of the past ten days? _____

Number of days I laughed: _____

Goal I want to set for the next 10 days: _____

Person/people who did or
said something to help me heal: _____

Anything else I have noticed
or want to remember/record: _____

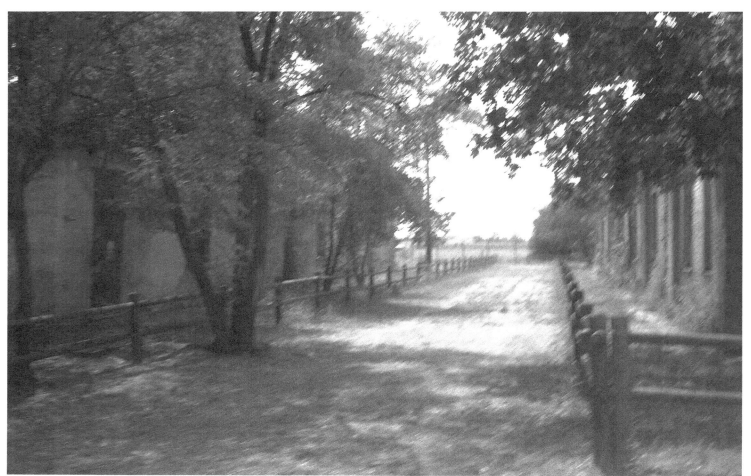

©STEPHEN RAINEY

> "*It is the bare courage to admit your weakness that makes you so strong.*"
> —CAROLYN MATHEWS LONG

What weakness are you willing to admit to? _____

The best part of my day: _____

Something that made me laugh: _____

Whom did I let "off the hook" today? _____

Someone / Something that brings me joy: _____

Where kindness touched my world today: _____

How I nourished my mind, body or spirit: _____

Number of hours I rested or slept in past 24 hours:
___ Rest   ___ Sleep

Prayer/Meditation for the day:
☼ Yes   ☼ No

I am grateful for: _____

Today I did this one little thing
    For the earth...
        for a friend or a stranger...
           for someone older or younger...
               for someone sicker...
                  in more need... _____

April 22ND

"I have a disease, but I also have a lot of other things."
—TERI GARR

What else I have: _____

The best part of my day: _____

Something that made me laugh: _____

Whom did I let "off the hook" today? _____

Someone / Something that brings me joy: _____

Where kindness touched my world today: _____

How I nourished my mind, body or spirit: _____

Number of hours I rested or slept in past 24 hours:
___ Rest   ___ Sleep

Prayer/Meditation for the day:
☼ Yes   ☼ No

I am grateful for: _____

Today I did this one little thing
    For the earth...
        for a friend or a stranger...
            for someone older or younger...
                for someone sicker...
                    in more need... _____

April 23RD

" To choose is also to begin. "
—STARHAWK

I choose: _____

The best part of my day: _____

Something that made me laugh: _____

Whom did I let "off the hook" today? _____

Someone / Something that brings me joy: _____

Where kindness touched my world today: _____

How I nourished my mind, body or spirit: _____

Number of hours I rested or slept in past 24 hours:
____Rest   ____Sleep

Prayer/Meditation for the day:
☼ Yes   ☼ No

I am grateful for: _____

Today I did this one little thing
    For the earth...
        for a friend or a stranger...
            for someone older or younger...
                for someone sicker...
                    in more need... _____

April 24TH

" Determination, patience and courage
are the only things needed to improve any
situation. "

—ANONYMOUS

I need more: _____

The best part of my day: _____

Something that made me laugh: _____

Whom did I let "off the hook" today? _____

Someone / Something that brings me joy: _____

Where kindness touched my world today: _____

How I nourished my mind, body or spirit: _____

Number of hours I rested or slept in past 24 hours:
___ Rest ___ Sleep

Prayer/Meditation for the day:
☼ Yes ☼ No

I am grateful for: _____

Today I did this one little thing
    For the earth...
        for a friend or a stranger...
            for someone older or younger...
                for someone sicker...
                    in more need... _____

> **❝** *There are times in life when joy comes to us in the purest form. When it is not tinged with fear or worry or sadness. These are the moments that we cling to. We embrace the present and we believe that there is nothing that can or will ever diminish this unbridled joy.* **❞**
>
> —JEANNE SELANDER MILLER
> *A BREATH AWAY*

How do I experience joy? _____

The best part of my day: _____

Something that made me laugh: _____

Whom did I let "off the hook" today? _____

Someone / Something that brings me joy: _____

Where kindness touched my world today: _____

How I nourished my mind, body or spirit: _____

Number of hours I rested or slept in past 24 hours:
____ Rest ____ Sleep

Prayer/Meditation for the day:
☀ Yes ☀ No

I am grateful for: _____

Today I did this one little thing
    For the earth...
        for a friend or a stranger...
            for someone older or younger...
                for someone sicker...
                    in more need... _____

April 26TH

" It does not do to dwell on dreams and forget to live."
—J.K. ROWLING

How I am remembering to live in today: _____

The best part of my day: _____

Something that made me laugh: _____

Whom did I let "off the hook" today? _____

Someone / Something that brings me joy: _____

Where kindness touched my world today: _____

How I nourished my mind, body or spirit: _____

Number of hours I rested or slept in past 24 hours:
___ Rest   ___ Sleep

Prayer/Meditation for the day:
☼ Yes   ☼ No

I am grateful for: _____

Today I did this one little thing
    For the earth...
        for a friend or a stranger...
           for someone older or younger...
               for someone sicker...
                  in more need... _____

" It seems to me that a pearl of a day like this, when the blossoms are out and the winds don't know where to blow from next for sheer crazy delight must be pretty near as good as heaven. "
—LUCY MAUD MONTGOMERY

Did I feel a breeze today? _____

The best part of my day: _____

Something that made me laugh: _____

Whom did I let "off the hook" today? _____

Someone / Something that brings me joy: _____

Where kindness touched my world today: _____

How I nourished my mind, body or spirit: _____

Number of hours I rested or slept in past 24 hours:
___ Rest   ___ Sleep

Prayer/Meditation for the day:
☼ Yes   ☼ No

I am grateful for: _____

Today I did this one little thing
 For the earth...
  for a friend or a stranger...
   for someone older or younger...
    for someone sicker...
     in more need... _____

April 28TH

" *You can close your eyes to reality but not to memories.* **"**
—STANISLAW JERZY LEC

I remember: _____

The best part of my day: _____

Something that made me laugh: _____

Whom did I let "off the hook" today? _____

Someone / Something that brings me joy: _____

Where kindness touched my world today: _____

How I nourished my mind, body or spirit: _____

Number of hours I rested or slept in past 24 hours:
___ Rest ___ Sleep

Prayer/Meditation for the day:
☼ Yes ☼ No

I am grateful for: _____

Today I did this one little thing
    For the earth...
        for a friend or a stranger...
            for someone older or younger...
                for someone sicker...
                    in more need... _____

> *"Let us be grateful to people who make us happy, they are the charming gardeners who make our souls blossom."*
> —MARCEL PROUST

Who helps my soul blossom: _____

The best part of my day: _____

Something that made me laugh: _____

Whom did I let "off the hook" today? _____

Someone / Something that brings me joy: _____

Where kindness touched my world today: _____

How I nourished my mind, body or spirit: _____

Number of hours I rested or slept in past 24 hours:
___Rest   ___Sleep

Prayer/Meditation for the day:
☼ Yes   ☼ No

I am grateful for: _____

Today I did this one little thing
   For the earth...
      for a friend or a stranger...
         for someone older or younger...
           for someone sicker...
             in more need... _____

April 30TH

> " *The best portion of a good man's life: his little,
> nameless unremembered acts of kindness and love.* "
> —WILLIAM WORDSWORTH

What small act of kindness
and love have I given this week? _____

The best part of my day: _____

Something that made me laugh: _____

Whom did I let "off the hook" today? _____

Someone / Something that brings me joy: _____

Where kindness touched my world today: _____

How I nourished my mind, body or spirit: _____

Number of hours I rested or slept in past 24 hours:
____ Rest   ____ Sleep

Prayer/Meditation for the day:
☼ Yes   ☼ No

I am grateful for: _____

Today I did this one little thing
    For the earth...
        for a friend or a stranger...
            for someone older or younger...
                for someone sicker...
                    in more need... _____

End of Month Review

Best part of the past ten days? _____

Number of days I laughed: _____

Goal I want to set for the next 10 days: _____

Person/people who did or
said something to help me heal: _____

Anything else I have noticed
or want to remember/record: _____

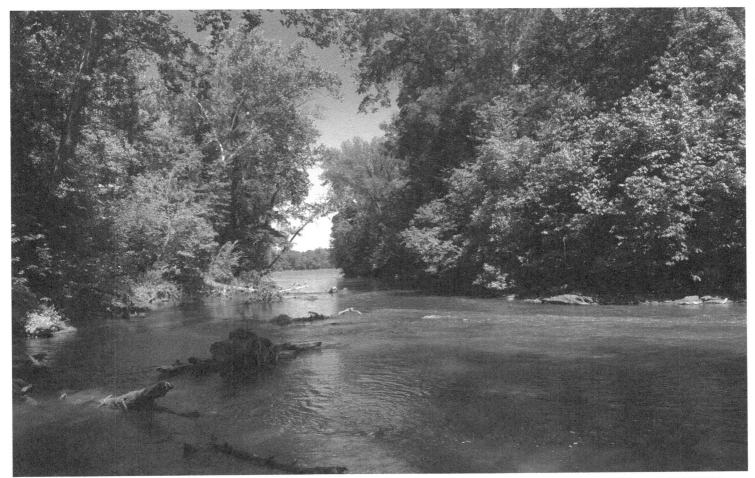

©NULLIE STOCKTON

May 1st

" We are all born with assignments, and when we discover what it is, our entire life will shift, change, and re-arrange. Our mindset will no longer focus on superficial tangible things. Our attitude, outlook, perspective, and energy level will shift. We no longer have the victim mentality. We suddenly realize why all the painful life experiences happened in their sequential order. The puzzle pieces will begin to align and the image and vision for your life will become clear. "
—CATHY HOLLOWAY HILL

My vision for my life: _____

The best part of my day: _____

Something that made me laugh: _____

Whom did I let "off the hook" today? _____

Someone / Something that brings me joy: _____

Where kindness touched my world today: _____

How I nourished my mind, body or spirit: _____

Number of hours I rested or slept in past 24 hours:
___ Rest ___ Sleep

Prayer/Meditation for the day:
☼ Yes ☼ No

I am grateful for: _____

Today I did this one little thing
   For the earth...
      for a friend or a stranger...
         for someone older or younger...
            for someone sicker...
               in more need... _____

> *"Watch your thoughts, for they become words. Watch your words, for they become actions. Watch your actions, for they become habits. Watch your habits, for they become character. Watch your character, for it becomes your destiny."*
> —ANONYMOUS

Today, I focused on: _____

The best part of my day: _____

Something that made me laugh: _____

Whom did I let "off the hook" today? _____

Someone / Something that brings me joy: _____

Where kindness touched my world today: _____

How I nourished my mind, body or spirit: _____

Number of hours I rested or slept in past 24 hours:
___Rest   ___Sleep

Prayer/Meditation for the day:
☼ Yes   ☼ No

I am grateful for: _____

Today I did this one little thing
    For the earth...
        for a friend or a stranger...
           for someone older or younger...
               for someone sicker...
                  in more need... _____

May 3RD

" Perhaps when we're forced to forfeit what we own, we lose any sentimental associations. Perhaps pawning our valuables frees us in the same way a house fire destroys not only our worldly goods, but our attachment to what's gone."

—SUE GRAFTON
V IS FOR VENGEANCE

What do I need to forfeit today? _____

The best part of my day: _____

Something that made me laugh: _____

Whom did I let "off the hook" today? _____

Someone / Something that brings me joy: _____

Where kindness touched my world today: _____

How I nourished my mind, body or spirit: _____

Number of hours I rested or slept in past 24 hours:
___ Rest   ___ Sleep

Prayer/Meditation for the day:
☼ Yes   ☼ No

I am grateful for: _____

Today I did this one little thing
    For the earth...
        for a friend or a stranger...
            for someone older or younger...
                for someone sicker...
                    in more need... _____

> " *You can feel that freedom and fulfillment that we all crave once you begin being honest with yourself, owning your desires and speaking them into existence.* "
>
> —ROBIN SHIRLEY
> WWW.ROBINSHIRLEY.COM

Where I saw grace today: _____

The best part of my day: _____

Something that made me laugh: _____

Whom did I let "off the hook" today? _____

Someone / Something that brings me joy: _____

Where kindness touched my world today: _____

How I nourished my mind, body or spirit: _____

Number of hours I rested or slept in past 24 hours:
____ Rest   ____ Sleep

Prayer/Meditation for the day:
☼ Yes   ☼ No

I am grateful for: _____

Today I did this one little thing
　　For the earth...
　　　　for a friend or a stranger...
　　　　　　for someone older or younger...
　　　　　　　　for someone sicker...
　　　　　　　　　　in more need... _____

May 5TH

"Fear can keep us up all night long, but faith makes one fine pillow."
—MARY MANIN MORRISSEY

How faith in my deepest experiences
has made my life brighter or easier: _____

The best part of my day: _____

Something that made me laugh: _____

Whom did I let "off the hook" today? _____

Someone / Something that brings me joy: _____

Where kindness touched my world today: _____

How I nourished my mind, body or spirit: _____

Number of hours I rested or slept in past 24 hours:
___Rest ___Sleep

Prayer/Meditation for the day:
☼ Yes ☼ No

I am grateful for: _____

Today I did this one little thing
    For the earth...
        for a friend or a stranger...
           for someone older or younger...
               for someone sicker...
                  in more need... _____

"Some days life breaks your heart with all that is hard: injustice, illness, injury, poverty, violence... But there is also courtesy, caring, kindness, generosity, connection, and incredible beauty. I think some force - the Great Mystery- conspired to show me the simple healing magic of everyday life, the beauty that reminds of us of our wholeness every day. And I am filled with gratitude, carried by grace."

—ORIAH

I see magic in: _____

The best part of my day: _____

Something that made me laugh: _____

Whom did I let "off the hook" today? _____

Someone / Something that brings me joy: _____

Where kindness touched my world today: _____

How I nourished my mind, body or spirit: _____

Number of hours I rested or slept in past 24 hours:
____Rest   ____Sleep

Prayer/Meditation for the day:
☀ Yes   ☀ No

I am grateful for: _____

Today I did this one little thing
    For the earth...
        for a friend or a stranger...
            for someone older or younger...
                for someone sicker...
                    in more need... _____

May 7TH

" *The view, though. The view. It is undeniably exhilarating.* "
—ANITA SHREVE
LIGHT ON SNOW

What view do I find exhilerating? _____

The best part of my day: _____

Something that made me laugh: _____

Whom did I let "off the hook" today? _____

Someone / Something that brings me joy: _____

Where kindness touched my world today: _____

How I nourished my mind, body or spirit: _____

Number of hours I rested or slept in past 24 hours:
____ Rest   ____ Sleep

Prayer/Meditation for the day:
☼ Yes   ☼ No

I am grateful for: _____

Today I did this one little thing
    For the earth...
        for a friend or a stranger...
           for someone older or younger...
             for someone sicker...
                in more need... _____

May 8TH

> "*When we feel pain from our physical disability, that pain amplifies our sense of hopelessness; the less hopeful we feel, the fewer endorphin and enkephalins and the more CCK we release. The more pain we experience due to these neurochemicals, the less able we are to feel hope. To break this cycle is key.*"
>
> —JEROME GROOPMAN
> *THE ANATOMY OF HOPE*

I am hopeful about: _____

The best part of my day: _____

Something that made me laugh: _____

Whom did I let "off the hook" today? _____

Someone / Something that brings me joy: _____

Where kindness touched my world today: _____

How I nourished my mind, body or spirit: _____

Number of hours I rested or slept in past 24 hours:
____Rest   ____Sleep

Prayer/Meditation for the day:
☼ Yes   ☼ No

I am grateful for: _____

Today I did this one little thing
    For the earth...
        for a friend or a stranger...
            for someone older or younger...
                for someone sicker...
                    in more need... _____

May 9TH

> **"** *"But man is not made for defeat," he said. "A man can be destroyed but not defeated.* **"**
> —ERNEST HEMINGWAY

What view do I find exhilerating? _____

The best part of my day: _____

Something that made me laugh: _____

Whom did I let "off the hook" today? _____

Someone / Something that brings me joy: _____

Where kindness touched my world today: _____

How I nourished my mind, body or spirit: _____

Number of hours I rested or slept in past 24 hours:
___ Rest   ___ Sleep

Prayer/Meditation for the day:
☼ Yes   ☼ No

I am grateful for: _____

Today I did this one little thing
    For the earth...
        for a friend or a stranger...
            for someone older or younger...
                for someone sicker...
                    in more need... _____

May 10ᵀᴴ

> " *Fighting grief is like struggling against an amorous gorilla—better to just get it over with.* "
> —DAN SHEEHAN
> *AFTER ACTION*

Something I did to nurture my soul: _____

The best part of my day: _____

Something that made me laugh: _____

Whom did I let "off the hook" today? _____

Someone / Something that brings me joy: _____

Where kindness touched my world today: _____

How I nourished my mind, body or spirit: _____

Number of hours I rested or slept in past 24 hours:
___ Rest   ___ Sleep

Prayer/Meditation for the day:
☼ Yes   ☼ No

I am grateful for: _____

Today I did this one little thing
    For the earth...
        for a friend or a stranger...
            for someone older or younger...
                for someone sicker...
                    in more need... _____

Early Month
Review

Best part of the past ten days? _____

Number of days I laughed: _____

Goal I want to set for the next 10 days: _____

Person/people who did or
said something to help me heal: _____

Anything else I have noticed
or want to remember/record: _____

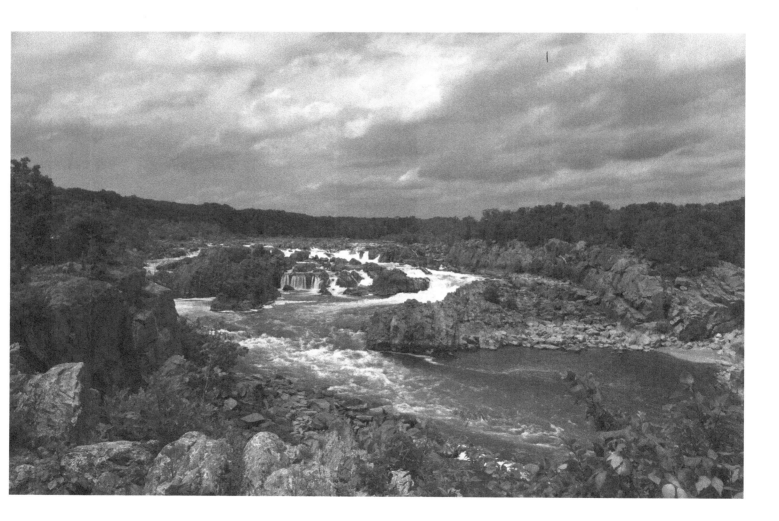

"Laughter is the tonic, the relief, the surcease for pain."
—CHARLIE CHAPLIN

I feel relieved when: _____

The best part of my day: _____

Something that made me laugh: _____

Whom did I let "off the hook" today? _____

Someone / Something that brings me joy: _____

Where kindness touched my world today: _____

How I nourished my mind, body or spirit: _____

Number of hours I rested or slept in past 24 hours:
___ Rest   ___ Sleep

Prayer/Meditation for the day:
☼ Yes   ☼ No

I am grateful for: _____

Today I did this one little thing
    For the earth...
        for a friend or a stranger...
           for someone older or younger...
              for someone sicker...
                in more need... _____

May 12TH

"When you hear the word 'disabled,' people immediately think about people who can't walk or talk or do everything that people take for granted. Now, I take nothing for granted. But I find the real disability is people who can't find joy in life and are bitter."

—TERI GARR

I find joy in: _____

The best part of my day: _____

Something that made me laugh: _____

Whom did I let "off the hook" today? _____

Someone / Something that brings me joy: _____

Where kindness touched my world today: _____

How I nourished my mind, body or spirit: _____

Number of hours I rested or slept in past 24 hours:
___ Rest ___ Sleep

Prayer/Meditation for the day:
☼ Yes ☼ No

I am grateful for: _____

Today I did this one little thing
   For the earth...
      for a friend or a stranger...
         for someone older or younger...
           for someone sicker...
              in more need... _____

"Every moment happens twice: inside and outside, and they are two different histories."
—ZADIE SMITH

A moment I had recently with two histories: _____

The best part of my day: _____

Something that made me laugh: _____

Whom did I let "off the hook" today? _____

Someone / Something that brings me joy: _____

Where kindness touched my world today: _____

How I nourished my mind, body or spirit: _____

Number of hours I rested or slept in past 24 hours:
___ Rest ___ Sleep

Prayer/Meditation for the day:
☼ Yes   ☼ No

I am grateful for: _____

Today I did this one little thing
　　For the earth...
　　　　for a friend or a stranger...
　　　　　　for someone older or younger...
　　　　　　　　for someone sicker...
　　　　　　　　　　in more need... _____

May 14TH

"*All that we are is the result of what we have thought.*"
—BUDDHA

I want to be free of: _____

The best part of my day: _____

Something that made me laugh: _____

Whom did I let "off the hook" today? _____

Someone / Something that brings me joy: _____

Where kindness touched my world today: _____

How I nourished my mind, body or spirit: _____

Number of hours I rested or slept in past 24 hours:
___ Rest   ___ Sleep

Prayer/Meditation for the day:
☼ Yes   ☼ No

I am grateful for: _____

Today I did this one little thing
    For the earth...
        for a friend or a stranger...
           for someone older or younger...
               for someone sicker...
                  in more need... _____

"Life is a great big canvas, and you should throw all the paint you can on it."
—DANNY KAYE

Today I created: _____

The best part of my day: _____

Something that made me laugh: _____

Whom did I let "off the hook" today? _____

Someone / Something that brings me joy: _____

Where kindness touched my world today: _____

How I nourished my mind, body or spirit: _____

Number of hours I rested or slept in past 24 hours:
____ Rest ____ Sleep

Prayer/Meditation for the day:
☼ Yes ☼ No

I am grateful for: _____

Today I did this one little thing
    For the earth...
        for a friend or a stranger...
           for someone older or younger...
             for someone sicker...
                in more need... _____

May 16TH

"Love may forgive all infirmities and love still in spite of them: but Love cannot cease to will their removal."
— C.S. LEWIS

I am inspired by: _____

The best part of my day: _____

Something that made me laugh: _____

Whom did I let "off the hook" today? _____

Someone / Something that brings me joy: _____

Where kindness touched my world today: _____

How I nourished my mind, body or spirit: _____

Number of hours I rested or slept in past 24 hours:
___ Rest   ___ Sleep

Prayer/Meditation for the day:
☼ Yes   ☼ No

I am grateful for: _____

Today I did this one little thing
    For the earth...
        for a friend or a stranger...
           for someone older or younger...
             for someone sicker...
                in more need... _____

" *The more you try to avoid suffering, the more you suffer, because smaller and more insignificant things begin to torture you, in proportion to your fear of being hurt. The one who does most to avoid suffering is, in the end, the one who suffers most.* "
—THOMAS MERTON

Am I afraid of being hurt? _____

The best part of my day: _____

Something that made me laugh: _____

Whom did I let "off the hook" today? _____

Someone / Something that brings me joy: _____

Where kindness touched my world today: _____

How I nourished my mind, body or spirit: _____

Number of hours I rested or slept in past 24 hours:
____Rest   ____Sleep

Prayer/Meditation for the day:
☼ Yes   ☼ No

I am grateful for: _____

Today I did this one little thing
    For the earth...
        for a friend or a stranger...
            for someone older or younger...
                for someone sicker...
                    in more need... _____

May 18ᵀᴴ

" When a person doesn't have gratitude, something is missing in his or her humanity. A person can almost be defined by his or her attitude toward gratitude. **"**
—ELIE WIESEL

I am grateful for: _____

The best part of my day: _____

Something that made me laugh: _____

Whom did I let "off the hook" today? _____

Someone / Something that brings me joy: _____

Where kindness touched my world today: _____

How I nourished my mind, body or spirit: _____

Number of hours I rested or slept in past 24 hours:
___Rest ___Sleep

Prayer/Meditation for the day:
☀ Yes   ☀ No

I am grateful for: _____

Today I did this one little thing
    For the earth...
        for a friend or a stranger...
            for someone older or younger...
                for someone sicker...
                    in more need... _____

" *Until you heal the wounds of your past, you are going to bleed. You can bandage the bleeding with food, with alcohol, with drugs, with work, with cigarettes, with sex; But eventually, it will all ooze through and stain your life. You must find the strength to open the wounds, stick your hands inside, pull out the core of the pain that is holding you in your past, the memories and make peace with them.* "

—IYANLA VANZANT
YESTERDAY, I CRIED

A memory I made peace with: _____

The best part of my day: _____

Something that made me laugh: _____

Whom did I let "off the hook" today? _____

Someone / Something that brings me joy: _____

Where kindness touched my world today: _____

How I nourished my mind, body or spirit: _____

Number of hours I rested or slept in past 24 hours:
___ Rest   ___ Sleep

Prayer/Meditation for the day:
☼ Yes   ☼ No

I am grateful for: _____

Today I did this one little thing
    For the earth...
        for a friend or a stranger...
            for someone older or younger...
                for someone sicker...
                    in more need... _____

May 20TH

Am I afraid of being hurt? _____

The best part of my day: _____

Something that made me laugh: _____

Whom did I let "off the hook" today? _____

Someone / Something that brings me joy: _____

Where kindness touched my world today: _____

How I nourished my mind, body or spirit: _____

Number of hours I rested or slept in past 24 hours:
____ Rest   ____ Sleep

Prayer/Meditation for the day:
☼ Yes   ☼ No

I am grateful for: _____

Today I did this one little thing
 For the earth...
  for a friend or a stranger...
   for someone older or younger...
    for someone sicker...
     in more need... _____

Mid Month Review

Best part of the past ten days? _____

Number of days I laughed: _____

Goal I want to set for the next 10 days: _____

Person/people who did or
said something to help me heal: _____

Anything else I have noticed
or want to remember/record: _____

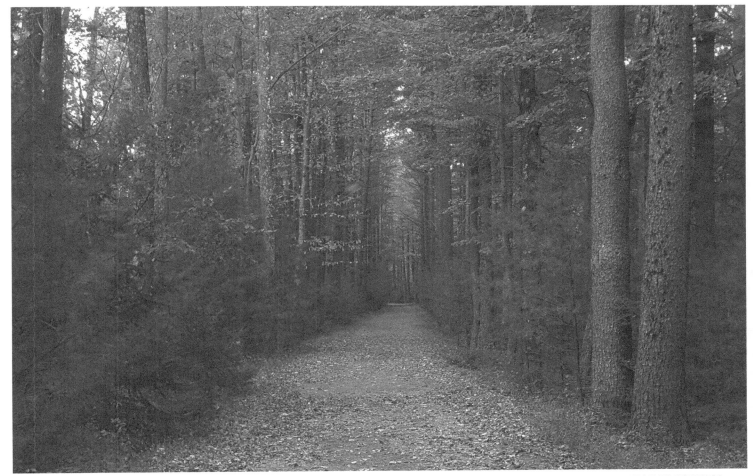

©NANCY CONNELL

May 21ST

" *Be comforted, dear soul! There is always light behind the clouds.* **"**
—LOUISA MAY ALCOTT

Where I saw some light today: _____

The best part of my day: _____

Something that made me laugh: _____

Whom did I let "off the hook" today? _____

Someone / Something that brings me joy: _____

Where kindness touched my world today: _____

How I nourished my mind, body or spirit: _____

Number of hours I rested or slept in past 24 hours:
___ Rest   ___ Sleep

Prayer/Meditation for the day:
☼ Yes   ☼ No

I am grateful for: _____

Today I did this one little thing
    For the earth...
        for a friend or a stranger...
            for someone older or younger...
                for someone sicker...
                    in more need... _____

" *All your life, you will be faced with a choice.*
You can choose love or hate... I choose love. **"**
—JOHNNY CASH

What choice am I making about my recovery? _____

The best part of my day: _____

Something that made me laugh: _____

Whom did I let "off the hook" today? _____

Someone / Something that brings me joy: _____

Where kindness touched my world today: _____

How I nourished my mind, body or spirit: _____

Number of hours I rested or slept in past 24 hours:
___ Rest   ___ Sleep

Prayer/Meditation for the day:
☼ Yes   ☼ No

I am grateful for: _____

Today I did this one little thing
    For the earth...
        for a friend or a stranger...
           for someone older or younger...
              for someone sicker...
                in more need... _____

May 23RD

" There are random moments - tossing a salad, coming up the driveway to the house, ironing the seams flat on a quilt square, standing at the kitchen window and looking out at the delphiniums, hearing a burst of laughter from one of my children's rooms - when I feel a wavelike rush of joy. This is my true religion: arbitrary moments of nearly painful happiness for a life I feel privileged to lead."

—ELIZABETH BERG
THE ART OF MENDING

One of my random moments: _____

The best part of my day: _____

Something that made me laugh: _____

Whom did I let "off the hook" today? _____

Someone / Something that brings me joy: _____

Where kindness touched my world today: _____

How I nourished my mind, body or spirit: _____

Number of hours I rested or slept in past 24 hours:
___ Rest   ___ Sleep

Prayer/Meditation for the day:
☼ Yes   ☼ No

I am grateful for: _____

Today I did this one little thing
    For the earth...
        for a friend or a stranger...
            for someone older or younger...
                for someone sicker...
                    in more need... _____

> "*Falling silent should be cultivated, the way the woods fall silent in the snow. Messages you can't send any other way can be heard.*"
> —PHYLLIS THEROUX

What I heard today: _____

The best part of my day: _____

Something that made me laugh: _____

Whom did I let "off the hook" today? _____

Someone / Something that brings me joy: _____

Where kindness touched my world today: _____

How I nourished my mind, body or spirit: _____

Number of hours I rested or slept in past 24 hours:
____ Rest   ____ Sleep

Prayer/Meditation for the day:
☼ Yes   ☼ No

I am grateful for: _____

Today I did this one little thing
     For the earth...
          for a friend or a stranger...
               for someone older or younger...
                    for someone sicker...
                         in more need... _____

May 25TH

"I was being asked to seek the miraculous in the ordinary and to wake up and recognize the extraordinary in this one precious life, as this life is short; don't waste it."
—JEANNE SELANDER MILLER
A BREATH AWAY

Where I found the miraculous in the ordinary: _____

The best part of my day: _____

Something that made me laugh: _____

Whom did I let "off the hook" today? _____

Someone / Something that brings me joy: _____

Where kindness touched my world today: _____

How I nourished my mind, body or spirit: _____

Number of hours I rested or slept in past 24 hours:
___ Rest   ___ Sleep

Prayer/Meditation for the day:
⚬ Yes   ⚬ No

I am grateful for: _____

Today I did this one little thing
    For the earth...
        for a friend or a stranger...
           for someone older or younger...
               for someone sicker...
                  in more need... _____

"*I will not allow myself to be less than I am to meet anyone's expectations.*"

—TERRI ST. CLOUD
BONESIGHARTS.COM

Something I love about myself: _____

The best part of my day: _____

Something that made me laugh: _____

Whom did I let "off the hook" today? _____

Someone / Something that brings me joy: _____

Where kindness touched my world today: _____

How I nourished my mind, body or spirit: _____

Number of hours I rested or slept in past 24 hours:
___Rest ___Sleep

Prayer/Meditation for the day:
☼ Yes ☼ No

I am grateful for: _____

Today I did this one little thing
 For the earth...
  for a friend or a stranger...
   for someone older or younger...
    for someone sicker...
     in more need... _____

May 27TH

"Love isn't an act, it's a whole life."
— BRIAN MOORE

Am I living in love? _____

The best part of my day: _____

Something that made me laugh: _____

Whom did I let "off the hook" today? _____

Someone / Something that brings me joy: _____

Where kindness touched my world today: _____

How I nourished my mind, body or spirit: _____

Number of hours I rested or slept in past 24 hours:
___ Rest ___ Sleep

Prayer/Meditation for the day:
☼ Yes ☼ No

I am grateful for: _____

Today I did this one little thing
    For the earth...
        for a friend or a stranger...
           for someone older or younger...
               for someone sicker...
                  in more need... _____

"It's not the load that breaks you, it's the way you carry it."
—LENA HORNE

Am I letting others into my
life in a constructive way? _____

The best part of my day: _____

Something that made me laugh: _____

Whom did I let "off the hook" today? _____

Someone / Something that brings me joy: _____

Where kindness touched my world today: _____

How I nourished my mind, body or spirit: _____

Number of hours I rested or slept in past 24 hours:
____ Rest ____ Sleep

Prayer/Meditation for the day:
⚬ Yes ⚬ No

I am grateful for: _____

Today I did this one little thing
    For the earth...
        for a friend or a stranger...
            for someone older or younger...
                for someone sicker...
                    in more need... _____

May 29TH

" The problem with doing nothing is not knowing when you are finished. "
—NELSON DEMILLE

What I am doing now that I didn't do previously: _____

The best part of my day: _____

Something that made me laugh: _____

Whom did I let "off the hook" today? _____

Someone / Something that brings me joy: _____

Where kindness touched my world today: _____

How I nourished my mind, body or spirit: _____

Number of hours I rested or slept in past 24 hours:
___ Rest ___ Sleep

Prayer/Meditation for the day:
☼ Yes ☼ No

I am grateful for: _____

Today I did this one little thing
For the earth...
for a friend or a stranger...
for someone older or younger...
for someone sicker...
in more need... _____

" This journey had taught me to love differently and more completely. "
—JEANNE SELANDER MILLER
A BREATH AWAY

How I can love differently: _____

The best part of my day: _____

Something that made me laugh: _____

Whom did I let "off the hook" today? _____

Someone / Something that brings me joy: _____

Where kindness touched my world today: _____

How I nourished my mind, body or spirit: _____

Number of hours I rested or slept in past 24 hours:
____Rest   ____Sleep

Prayer/Meditation for the day:
☼ Yes   ☼ No

I am grateful for: _____

Today I did this one little thing
    For the earth...
        for a friend or a stranger...
            for someone older or younger...
                for someone sicker...
                    in more need... _____

May 31ST

" I prefer a church which is bruised, hurting and dirty because it
has been out on the streets, rather than a church which is unhealthy
from being confined and from clinging to its own security. **"**
—POPE FRANCIS

What community have I created
from my bruises and pain? _____

The best part of my day: _____

Something that made me laugh: _____

Whom did I let "off the hook" today? _____

Someone / Something that brings me joy: _____

Where kindness touched my world today: _____

How I nourished my mind, body or spirit: _____

Number of hours I rested or slept in past 24 hours:
___ Rest   ___ Sleep

Prayer/Meditation for the day:
☼ Yes   ☼ No

I am grateful for: _____

Today I did this one little thing
    For the earth...
        for a friend or a stranger...
            for someone older or younger...
                for someone sicker...
                    in more need... _____

End of Month Review

Best part of the past ten days? _____

Number of days I laughed: _____

Goal I want to set for the next 10 days: _____

Person/people who did or
said something to help me heal: _____

Anything else I have noticed
or want to remember/record: _____

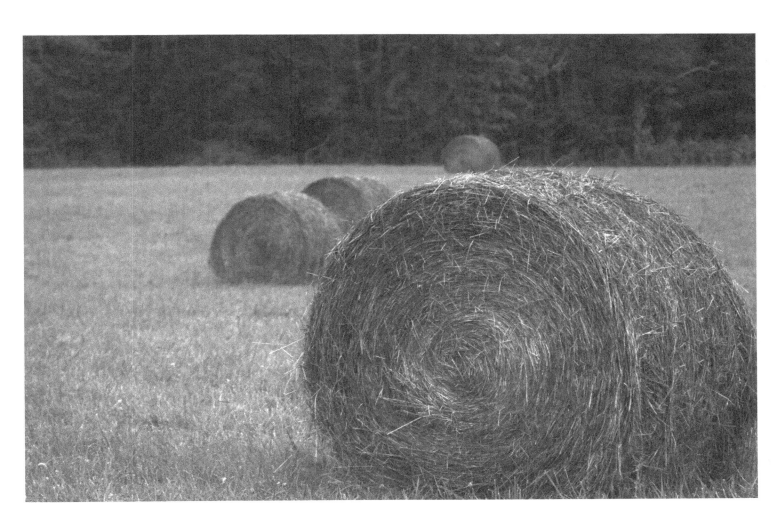

June 1ˢᵀ

> " *Tears are words waiting to be written.* "
> —PAULO COELHO

What have my tears said? _____

The best part of my day: _____

Something that made me laugh: _____

Whom did I let "off the hook" today? _____

Someone / Something that brings me joy: _____

Where kindness touched my world today: _____

How I nourished my mind, body or spirit: _____

Number of hours I rested or slept in past 24 hours:
___ Rest   ___ Sleep

Prayer/Meditation for the day:
☼ Yes   ☼ No

I am grateful for: _____

Today I did this one little thing
    For the earth...
        for a friend or a stranger...
            for someone older or younger...
                for someone sicker...
                    in more need... _____

"*Many persons have the wrong idea of what constitutes true happiness. It is not attained through self-gratification but through fidelity to a worthy purpose.*"
—HELEN KELLER

Do I want to be right or do I want to be happy? _____

The best part of my day: _____

Something that made me laugh: _____

Whom did I let "off the hook" today? _____

Someone / Something that brings me joy: _____

Where kindness touched my world today: _____

How I nourished my mind, body or spirit: _____

Number of hours I rested or slept in past 24 hours:
___Rest   ___Sleep

Prayer/Meditation for the day:
☼ Yes   ☼ No

I am grateful for: _____

Today I did this one little thing
 For the earth...
  for a friend or a stranger...
   for someone older or younger...
    for someone sicker...
     in more need... _____

June 3RD

*"Courage is not the absence of fear, but rather the
judgment that something else is more important than fear."*
—AMBROSE REDMOON

What am I willing to move forward
with, thus not allowing fear to overrule? _____

The best part of my day: _____

Something that made me laugh: _____

Whom did I let "off the hook" today? _____

Someone / Something that brings me joy: _____

Where kindness touched my world today: _____

How I nourished my mind, body or spirit: _____

Number of hours I rested or slept in past 24 hours:
___ Rest   ___ Sleep

Prayer/Meditation for the day:
☼ Yes   ☼ No

I am grateful for: _____

Today I did this one little thing
    For the earth...
        for a friend or a stranger...
            for someone older or younger...
                for someone sicker...
                    in more need... _____

June 4ᵀᴴ

❝*Sometimes all it takes is a tiny shift of perspective
to see something familiar in a totally new light.*❞

—DAN BROWN

FROM DIGITAL FORTRESS © 1998 BY DAN BROWN. REPRINTED BY
PERMISSION OF ST. MARTIN'S PRESS. ALL RIGHTS RESERVED.

What shift do I need to make? _____

The best part of my day: _____

Something that made me laugh: _____

Whom did I let "off the hook" today? _____

Someone / Something that brings me joy: _____

Where kindness touched my world today: _____

How I nourished my mind, body or spirit: _____

Number of hours I rested or slept in past 24 hours:
___ Rest ___ Sleep

Prayer/Meditation for the day:
☼ Yes ☼ No

I am grateful for: _____

Today I did this one little thing
    For the earth...
        for a friend or a stranger...
            for someone older or younger...
                for someone sicker...
                   in more need... _____

June 5TH

" Do what you can, with what you have, where you are. "
—THEODORE ROOSEVELT

Do I really believe that I
am enough just as I am? _____

The best part of my day: _____

Something that made me laugh: _____

Whom did I let "off the hook" today? _____

Someone / Something that brings me joy: _____

Where kindness touched my world today: _____

How I nourished my mind, body or spirit: _____

Number of hours I rested or slept in past 24 hours:
___Rest   ___Sleep

Prayer/Meditation for the day:
☀ Yes   ☀ No

I am grateful for: _____

Today I did this one little thing
    For the earth...
        for a friend or a stranger...
            for someone older or younger...
                for someone sicker...
                    in more need... _____

"Slowly I began to understand that the plans God has for us don't just include "good" things, but the whole array of human events... I remember my mom saying that many people look for miracles — things that in their human minds "fix" a difficult situation. Many miracles, however, are not a change to the normal course of human events; they're found in God's ability and desire to sustain and nurture people through even the worst situations. Somewhere along the way, I stopped demanding that God fix the problems in my life and started to be thankful for his presence as I endured them."

—LISA BEAMER

LET'S ROLL!: ORDINARY PEOPLE, EXTRAORDINARY COURAGE

Where have I seen God's presence? _____

The best part of my day: _____

Something that made me laugh: _____

Whom did I let "off the hook" today? _____

Someone / Something that brings me joy: _____

Where kindness touched my world today: _____

How I nourished my mind, body or spirit: _____

Number of hours I rested or slept in past 24 hours:
___ Rest ___ Sleep

Prayer/Meditation for the day:
☼ Yes ☼ No

I am grateful for: _____

Today I did this one little thing
    For the earth...
        for a friend or a stranger...
            for someone older or younger...
                for someone sicker...
                    in more need... _____

June 7TH

> *"Confront the dark parts of yourself, and work to banish them with illumination and forgiveness. Your willingness to wrestle with your demons will cause your angels to sing."*
> —AUGUST WILSON

I am willing to confront my: _____

The best part of my day: _____

Something that made me laugh: _____

Whom did I let "off the hook" today? _____

Someone / Something that brings me joy: _____

Where kindness touched my world today: _____

How I nourished my mind, body or spirit: _____

Number of hours I rested or slept in past 24 hours:
____Rest   ____Sleep

Prayer/Meditation for the day:
☼ Yes   ☼ No

I am grateful for: _____

Today I did this one little thing
   For the earth...
      for a friend or a stranger...
         for someone older or younger...
            for someone sicker...
               in more need... _____

"*It does not matter how slowly you go, as long as you don't stop.*"
—CONFUCIUS

Something / Someone I am energized by: _____

The best part of my day: _____

Something that made me laugh: _____

Whom did I let "off the hook" today? _____

Someone / Something that brings me joy: _____

Where kindness touched my world today: _____

How I nourished my mind, body or spirit: _____

Number of hours I rested or slept in past 24 hours:
___ Rest   ___ Sleep

Prayer/Meditation for the day:
☼ Yes   ☼ No

I am grateful for: _____

Today I did this one little thing
    For the earth...
        for a friend or a stranger...
            for someone older or younger...
                for someone sicker...
                    in more need... _____

June 9TH

" You have to bring joy back into your life because your soul dies if you don't have it. It's the evolution of the heart and compassion is what is missing technically. Humans have proceeded to technological advances before without heart balance, without heart evolution. And it has been disastrous. So we are here to evolve heart first until the heart is aligned with this knowledge."

—DOLORES CANNON
THE THREE WAVES OF VOLUNTEERS

Something that brought me joy: _____

The best part of my day: _____

Something that made me laugh: _____

Whom did I let "off the hook" today? _____

Someone / Something that brings me joy: _____

Where kindness touched my world today: _____

How I nourished my mind, body or spirit: _____

Number of hours I rested or slept in past 24 hours:
____ Rest   ____ Sleep

Prayer/Meditation for the day:
☼ Yes   ☼ No

I am grateful for: _____

Today I did this one little thing
    For the earth...
        for a friend or a stranger...
            for someone older or younger...
                for someone sicker...
                    in more need... _____

June 10TH

" If it does not support your soul, it's time to let it go. "
— BARRY DENNIS
AUTHOR, TITLE, COPYRIGHT, HAY HOUSE INC, CARLSBAD, CA

Something I want to let go of: _____

The best part of my day: _____

Something that made me laugh: _____

Whom did I let "off the hook" today? _____

Someone / Something that brings me joy: _____

Where kindness touched my world today: _____

How I nourished my mind, body or spirit: _____

Number of hours I rested or slept in past 24 hours:
___ Rest   ___ Sleep

Prayer/Meditation for the day:
☼ Yes   ☼ No

I am grateful for: _____

Today I did this one little thing
    For the earth...
        for a friend or a stranger...
           for someone older or younger...
              for someone sicker...
                in more need... _____

Early Month Review

Best part of the past ten days? _____

Number of days I laughed: _____

Goal I want to set for the next 10 days: _____

Person/people who did or
said something to help me heal: _____

Anything else I have noticed
or want to remember/record: _____

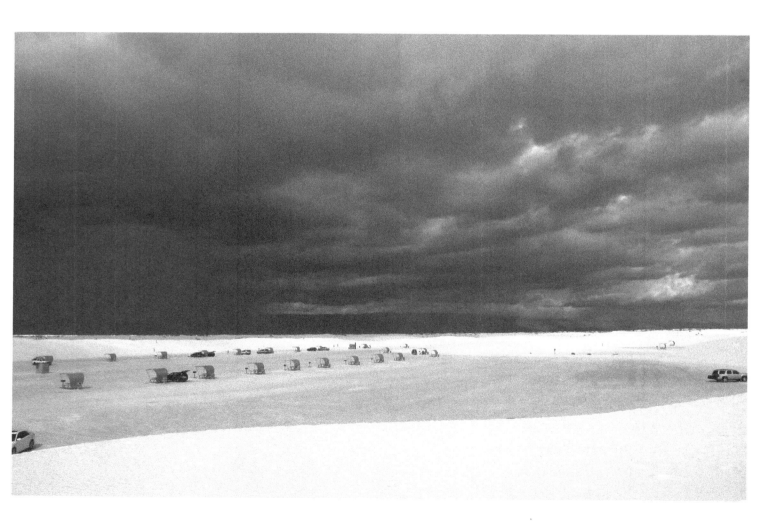

"If the only prayer you said in your whole life was, "thank you," that would suffice."
—MEISTER ECKHART

I said Thank You to/for: _____

The best part of my day: _____

Something that made me laugh: _____

Whom did I let "off the hook" today? _____

Someone / Something that brings me joy: _____

Where kindness touched my world today: _____

How I nourished my mind, body or spirit: _____

Number of hours I rested or slept in past 24 hours:
___ Rest ___ Sleep

Prayer/Meditation for the day:
☼ Yes ☼ No

I am grateful for: _____

Today I did this one little thing
    For the earth...
        for a friend or a stranger...
            for someone older or younger...
                for someone sicker...
                    in more need... _____

June 12TH

" There's a limit to how much one can help others - the balance
point is defined by when it does not compromise you and your
ability to help yourself, your family, and others in need. "
—B. ROBERT MOZAYENI, MD

Have I found my balance point yet? _____

The best part of my day: _____

Something that made me laugh: _____

Whom did I let "off the hook" today? _____

Someone / Something that brings me joy: _____

Where kindness touched my world today: _____

How I nourished my mind, body or spirit: _____

Number of hours I rested or slept in past 24 hours:
____ Rest ____ Sleep

Prayer/Meditation for the day:
☼ Yes   ☼ No

I am grateful for: _____

Today I did this one little thing
     For the earth...
          for a friend or a stranger...
               for someone older or younger...
                    for someone sicker...
                         in more need... _____

" It's just my job to notice my emptiness and find graceful ways to live as a broken, unfilled human—and maybe to help myself and others feel a teeny bit better. "

—GLENNON DOYLE MELTON

CARRY ON, WARRIOR: THE POWER OF EMBRACING YOUR MESSY, BEAUTIFUL LIFE

How I am helping myself and others
even as a broken, unfilled human: _____

The best part of my day: _____

Something that made me laugh: _____

Whom did I let "off the hook" today? _____

Someone / Something that brings me joy: _____

Where kindness touched my world today: _____

How I nourished my mind, body or spirit: _____

Number of hours I rested or slept in past 24 hours:
____ Rest   ____ Sleep

Prayer/Meditation for the day:
☼ Yes   ☼ No

I am grateful for: _____

Today I did this one little thing
    For the earth...
        for a friend or a stranger...
            for someone older or younger...
                for someone sicker...
                    in more need... _____

June 14TH

"To send a letter is a good way to go somewhere without moving anything but your heart."
—PHYLLIS THEROUX

How will I move my heart today? _____

The best part of my day: _____

Something that made me laugh: _____

Whom did I let "off the hook" today? _____

Someone / Something that brings me joy: _____

Where kindness touched my world today: _____

How I nourished my mind, body or spirit: _____

Number of hours I rested or slept in past 24 hours:
___ Rest   ___ Sleep

Prayer/Meditation for the day:
☼ Yes   ☼ No

I am grateful for: _____

Today I did this one little thing
　　For the earth...
　　　　for a friend or a stranger...
　　　　　　for someone older or younger...
　　　　　　　　for someone sicker...
　　　　　　　　　　in more need... _____

June 15ᵀᴴ

> *" The unendurable is the beginning of the curve of joy. "*
> —DJUNA BARNES

Can I see the beginning of the curve? _____

The best part of my day: _____

Something that made me laugh: _____

Whom did I let "off the hook" today? _____

Someone / Something that brings me joy: _____

Where kindness touched my world today: _____

How I nourished my mind, body or spirit: _____

Number of hours I rested or slept in past 24 hours:
___ Rest   ___ Sleep

Prayer/Meditation for the day:
☼ Yes   ☼ No

I am grateful for: _____

Today I did this one little thing
    For the earth...
        for a friend or a stranger...
           for someone older or younger...
              for someone sicker...
                in more need... _____

June 16TH

" The more isolated and disconnected we are, the more shattered and distorted our self-identity. We are not healthy when we are alone. We find ourselves when we connect to others. Without community we don't know who we are. [...] When we live outside of healthy community, we not only lose others, we lose ourselves. [...] Who we understand ourselves to be is dramatically affected for better or worse by those we hold closest to us. "

—ERWIN RAPHAEL MCMANUS
SOUL CRAVINGS: AN EXPLORATION OF THE HUMAN SPIRIT

Whom did I connect with today? _____

The best part of my day: _____

Something that made me laugh: _____

Whom did I let "off the hook" today? _____

Someone / Something that brings me joy: _____

Where kindness touched my world today: _____

How I nourished my mind, body or spirit: _____

Number of hours I rested or slept in past 24 hours:
____Rest   ____Sleep

Prayer/Meditation for the day:
☼ Yes   ☼ No

I am grateful for: _____

Today I did this one little thing
    For the earth...
        for a friend or a stranger...
            for someone older or younger...
                for someone sicker...
                    in more need... _____

June 17TH

" Its so hard to talk when you want to kill yourself. That's above and beyond everything else, and it's not a mental complaint-it's a physical thing, like it's physically hard to open your mouth and make the words come out. They don't come out smooth and in conjunction with your brain the way normal people's words do; they come out in chunks as if from a crushed-ice dispenser; you stumble on them as they gather behind your lower lip. So you just keep quiet. "

—NED VIZZINI
IT'S KIND OF A FUNNY STORY

A time when I opened my
mouth and didn't keep quiet: _____

The best part of my day: _____

Something that made me laugh: _____

Whom did I let "off the hook" today? _____

Someone / Something that brings me joy: _____

Where kindness touched my world today: _____

How I nourished my mind, body or spirit: _____

Number of hours I rested or slept in past 24 hours:
____Rest   ____Sleep

Prayer/Meditation for the day:
☼ Yes   ☼ No

I am grateful for: _____

Today I did this one little thing
    For the earth...
        for a friend or a stranger...
           for someone older or younger...
               for someone sicker...
                  in more need... _____

June 18TH

*" When you can't make sense of something in your head,
make a peaceful space for it in your heart. And just be.*"
—CINDY FISCHTHAL

Today, I am holding _____ in my heart.

The best part of my day: _____

Something that made me laugh: _____

Whom did I let "off the hook" today? _____

Someone / Something that brings me joy: _____

Where kindness touched my world today: _____

How I nourished my mind, body or spirit: _____

Number of hours I rested or slept in past 24 hours:
___Rest   ___Sleep

Prayer/Meditation for the day:
☼ Yes   ☼ No

I am grateful for: _____

Today I did this one little thing
     For the earth...
          for a friend or a stranger...
               for someone older or younger...
                    for someone sicker...
                         in more need... _____

> " *But there is suffering in life, and there are defeats. No one can avoid them. But it's better to lose some of the battles in the struggles for your dreams than to be defeated without ever knowing what you're fighting for.* "
>
> —PAULO COELHO

A stressor I have removed from my life: _____

The best part of my day: _____

Something that made me laugh: _____

Whom did I let "off the hook" today? _____

Someone / Something that brings me joy: _____

Where kindness touched my world today: _____

How I nourished my mind, body or spirit: _____

Number of hours I rested or slept in past 24 hours:
___Rest   ___Sleep

Prayer/Meditation for the day:
☼ Yes   ☼ No

I am grateful for: _____

Today I did this one little thing
    For the earth...
        for a friend or a stranger...
            for someone older or younger...
                for someone sicker...
                    in more need... _____

June 20TH

"Anger is like flowing water; there's nothing wrong with it as long as you let it flow. Hate is like stagnant water; anger that you denied yourself the freedom to feel, the freedom to flow; water that you gathered in one place and left to forget. Stagnant water becomes dirty, stinky, disease-ridden, poisonous, deadly; that is your hate. On flowing water travels little paper boats; paper boats of forgiveness. Allow yourself to feel anger, allow your waters to flow, along with all the paper boats of forgiveness. Be human."

— C. JOYBELL

Something I need to let flow: _____

The best part of my day: _____

Something that made me laugh: _____

Whom did I let "off the hook" today? _____

Someone / Something that brings me joy: _____

Where kindness touched my world today: _____

How I nourished my mind, body or spirit: _____

Number of hours I rested or slept in past 24 hours:
___ Rest ___ Sleep

Prayer/Meditation for the day:
☼ Yes ☼ No

I am grateful for: _____

Today I did this one little thing
For the earth...
for a friend or a stranger...
for someone older or younger...
for someone sicker...
in more need... _____

Mid Month Review

Best part of the past ten days? _____

Number of days I laughed: _____

Goal I want to set for the next 10 days: _____

Person/people who did or
said something to help me heal: _____

Anything else I have noticed
or want to remember/record: _____

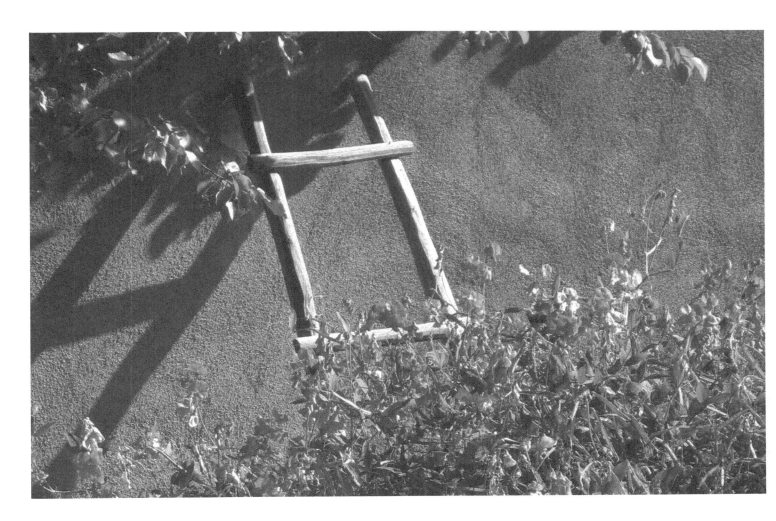

June 21ST

> **"***If you can take all the energy you are putting into getting well one day into your regular day life what would that look like?***"**
> —ANGELE RICE

What do I want my healed life to look like? _____

The best part of my day: _____

Something that made me laugh: _____

Whom did I let "off the hook" today? _____

Someone / Something that brings me joy: _____

Where kindness touched my world today: _____

How I nourished my mind, body or spirit: _____

Number of hours I rested or slept in past 24 hours:
___ Rest ___ Sleep

Prayer/Meditation for the day:
☼ Yes   ☼ No

I am grateful for: _____

Today I did this one little thing
    For the earth...
        for a friend or a stranger...
            for someone older or younger...
                for someone sicker...
                    in more need... _____

> **"** *Dreams are like stars... you may never touch them, but*
> *if you follow them they will lead you to your destiny.* **"**
> —ANONYMOUS

I dream of: _____

The best part of my day: _____

Something that made me laugh: _____

Whom did I let "off the hook" today? _____

Someone / Something that brings me joy: _____

Where kindness touched my world today: _____

How I nourished my mind, body or spirit: _____

Number of hours I rested or slept in past 24 hours:
___ Rest   ___ Sleep

Prayer/Meditation for the day:
☼ Yes   ☼ No

I am grateful for: _____

Today I did this one little thing
　　For the earth...
　　　　for a friend or a stranger...
　　　　　　for someone older or younger...
　　　　　　　　for someone sicker...
　　　　　　　　　　in more need... _____

June 23RD

"A fine glass vase goes from treasure to trash, the moment it is broken. Fortunately, something else happens to you and me. Pick up your pieces. Then, help me gather mine."
—VERA NAZARIAN

Whose pieces have I helped gather? _____

The best part of my day: _____

Something that made me laugh: _____

Whom did I let "off the hook" today? _____

Someone / Something that brings me joy: _____

Where kindness touched my world today: _____

How I nourished my mind, body or spirit: _____

Number of hours I rested or slept in past 24 hours:
____ Rest   ____ Sleep

Prayer/Meditation for the day:
☼ Yes   ☼ No

I am grateful for: _____

Today I did this one little thing
    For the earth...
        for a friend or a stranger...
            for someone older or younger...
                for someone sicker...
                    in more need... _____

> **"** *I believe that words are strong, that they can overwhelm*
> *what we fear when fear seems more awful than life is good.* **"**
> —ANDREW SOLOMON

Strong words that I connect with today: _____

The best part of my day: _____

Something that made me laugh: _____

Whom did I let "off the hook" today? _____

Someone / Something that brings me joy: _____

Where kindness touched my world today: _____

How I nourished my mind, body or spirit: _____

Number of hours I rested or slept in past 24 hours:
___ Rest   ___ Sleep

Prayer/Meditation for the day:
☼ Yes   ☼ No

I am grateful for: _____

Today I did this one little thing
    For the earth...
        for a friend or a stranger...
            for someone older or younger...
                for someone sicker...
                    in more need... _____

June 25TH

"I have been bent and broken, but - I hope - into a better shape."
—EMILY DICKINSON

What trials and tribulations have
made me who I am today? How have
they changed me into a better shape? _____

The best part of my day: _____

Something that made me laugh: _____

Whom did I let "off the hook" today? _____

Someone / Something that brings me joy: _____

Where kindness touched my world today: _____

How I nourished my mind, body or spirit: _____

Number of hours I rested or slept in past 24 hours:
___ Rest   ___ Sleep

Prayer/Meditation for the day:
☼ Yes   ☼ No

I am grateful for: _____

Today I did this one little thing
    For the earth...
        for a friend or a stranger...
           for someone older or younger...
              for someone sicker...
                in more need... _____

> " *To have a quiet mind is to possess one's mind
> wholly; to have a calm spirit is to possess one's self.* "
> —HAMILTON WRIGHT MABIE

Something that calmed me today: _____

The best part of my day: _____

Something that made me laugh: _____

Whom did I let "off the hook" today? _____

Someone / Something that brings me joy: _____

Where kindness touched my world today: _____

How I nourished my mind, body or spirit: _____

Number of hours I rested or slept in past 24 hours:
___ Rest   ___ Sleep

Prayer/Meditation for the day:
☼ Yes   ☼ No

I am grateful for: _____

Today I did this one little thing
    For the earth...
        for a friend or a stranger...
            for someone older or younger...
                for someone sicker...
                    in more need... _____

June 27TH

" It was a nugget way down deep. a lump of gold, her belief in herself, her self-love, her real. that's what she needed to focus on. grow that, and the rest would take care of itself. "
—TERRI ST. CLOUD
BONESIGHARTS.COM

I surrendered to: _____

The best part of my day: _____

Something that made me laugh: _____

Whom did I let "off the hook" today? _____

Someone / Something that brings me joy: _____

Where kindness touched my world today: _____

How I nourished my mind, body or spirit: _____

Number of hours I rested or slept in past 24 hours:
___ Rest ___ Sleep

Prayer/Meditation for the day:
☼ Yes ☼ No

I am grateful for: _____

Today I did this one little thing
For the earth...
for a friend or a stranger...
for someone older or younger...
for someone sicker...
in more need... _____

" *The sea does not reward those who are too anxious, too greedy, or too impatient. To dig for treasures shows not only impatience and greed, but lack of faith. Patience, patience, patience, is what the sea teaches. Patience and faith. One should lie empty, open, choiceless as a beach—waiting for a gift from the sea.* "
—ANNE MORROW LINDBERGH

I showed patience when: _____

The best part of my day: _____

Something that made me laugh: _____

Whom did I let "off the hook" today? _____

Someone / Something that brings me joy: _____

Where kindness touched my world today: _____

How I nourished my mind, body or spirit: _____

Number of hours I rested or slept in past 24 hours:
___ Rest ___ Sleep

Prayer/Meditation for the day:
☼ Yes ☼ No

I am grateful for: _____

Today I did this one little thing
For the earth...
for a friend or a stranger...
for someone older or younger...
for someone sicker...
in more need... _____

June 29TH

*"I was always looking outside myself for strength and
confidence but it comes from within. It is there all the time."*
—ANNA FREUD

Something I do well: _____

The best part of my day: _____

Something that made me laugh: _____

Whom did I let "off the hook" today? _____

Someone / Something that brings me joy: _____

Where kindness touched my world today: _____

How I nourished my mind, body or spirit: _____

Number of hours I rested or slept in past 24 hours:
____ Rest   ____ Sleep

Prayer/Meditation for the day:
☼ Yes   ☼ No

I am grateful for: _____

Today I did this one little thing
    For the earth...
        for a friend or a stranger...
            for someone older or younger...
                for someone sicker...
                    in more need... _____

"*Love doesn't make the world go round. Love is what makes the ride worthwhile.*"
—FRANKLIN P. JONES

I love: _____

The best part of my day: _____

Something that made me laugh: _____

Whom did I let "off the hook" today? _____

Someone / Something that brings me joy: _____

Where kindness touched my world today: _____

How I nourished my mind, body or spirit: _____

Number of hours I rested or slept in past 24 hours:
____Rest ____Sleep

Prayer/Meditation for the day:
☼ Yes ☼ No

I am grateful for: _____

Today I did this one little thing
   For the earth...
      for a friend or a stranger...
         for someone older or younger...
           for someone sicker...
              in more need... _____

End of Month Review

Best part of the past ten days? _____

Number of days I laughed: _____

Goal I want to set for the next 10 days: _____

Person/people who did or
said something to help me heal: _____

Anything else I have noticed
or want to remember/record: _____

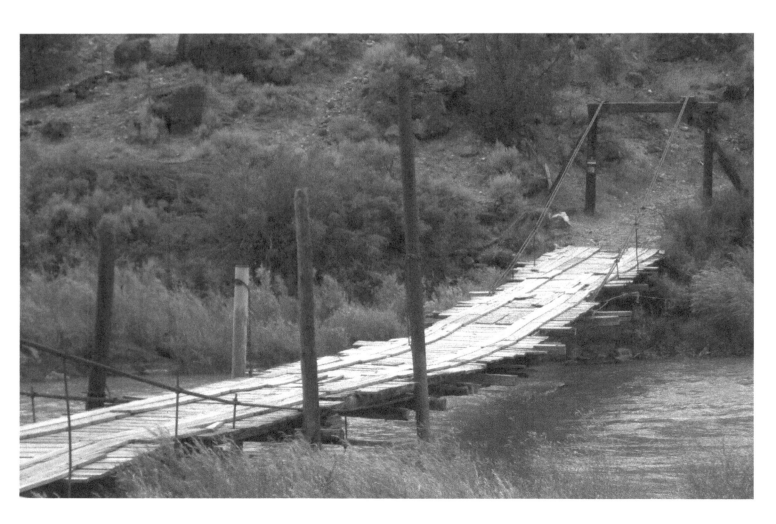

> **"***If you reveal who you truly are, you will attract***
> ***the people who will most complement your life.***"**
> —EL HAJI NERO

Who complemented my life today: _____

The best part of my day: _____

Something that made me laugh: _____

Whom did I let "off the hook" today? _____

Someone / Something that brings me joy: _____

Where kindness touched my world today: _____

How I nourished my mind, body or spirit: _____

Number of hours I rested or slept in past 24 hours:
___Rest   ___Sleep

Prayer/Meditation for the day:
☼ Yes   ☼ No

I am grateful for: _____

Today I did this one little thing
    For the earth...
        for a friend or a stranger...
            for someone older or younger...
                for someone sicker...
                    in more need... _____

July 2ND

" Do not fear the winds of adversity. Remember:
A kite rises against the wind rather than with it. "
—ANONYMOUS

I am ready to receive: _____

The best part of my day: _____

Something that made me laugh: _____

Whom did I let "off the hook" today? _____

Someone / Something that brings me joy: _____

Where kindness touched my world today: _____

How I nourished my mind, body or spirit: _____

Number of hours I rested or slept in past 24 hours:
___Rest   ___Sleep

Prayer/Meditation for the day:
☼ Yes   ☼ No

I am grateful for: _____

Today I did this one little thing
    For the earth...
        for a friend or a stranger...
            for someone older or younger...
                for someone sicker...
                    in more need... _____

"In seeking happiness for others, you find it for yourself."
—ANONYMOUS

The person I seek happiness for is: _____

The best part of my day: _____

Something that made me laugh: _____

Whom did I let "off the hook" today? _____

Someone / Something that brings me joy: _____

Where kindness touched my world today: _____

How I nourished my mind, body or spirit: _____

Number of hours I rested or slept in past 24 hours:
____Rest   ____Sleep

Prayer/Meditation for the day:
☼ Yes   ☼ No

I am grateful for: _____

Today I did this one little thing
    For the earth...
        for a friend or a stranger...
            for someone older or younger...
                for someone sicker...
                    in more need... _____

July 4ᵀᴴ

> " *Don't ever discount the wonder of your tears. They can be healing waters and a stream of joy. Sometimes they are the best words the heart can speak.* "
>
> —WM PAUL YOUNG
> *THE SHACK*

The last time I cried, my heart was saying: _____

The best part of my day: _____

Something that made me laugh: _____

Whom did I let "off the hook" today? _____

Someone / Something that brings me joy: _____

Where kindness touched my world today: _____

How I nourished my mind, body or spirit: _____

Number of hours I rested or slept in past 24 hours:
___ Rest   ___ Sleep

Prayer/Meditation for the day:
☼ Yes   ☼ No

I am grateful for: _____

Today I did this one little thing
　　For the earth...
　　　　for a friend or a stranger...
　　　　　　for someone older or younger...
　　　　　　　　for someone sicker...
　　　　　　　　　　in more need... _____

> *"Hold no grudges. Find no fault with others. DO show appreciation for all efforts, not only for self but appreciation for the OPPORTUNITY to speak to and with others as to how they should appreciate THEIR opportunities among their associates in WHATEVER walk of life it may be."*
> —EDGAR CAYCE

How did I show my appreciation today? _____

The best part of my day: _____

Something that made me laugh: _____

Whom did I let "off the hook" today? _____

Someone / Something that brings me joy: _____

Where kindness touched my world today: _____

How I nourished my mind, body or spirit: _____

Number of hours I rested or slept in past 24 hours:
___Rest ___Sleep

Prayer/Meditation for the day:
☼ Yes ☼ No

I am grateful for: _____

Today I did this one little thing
  For the earth...
    for a friend or a stranger...
      for someone older or younger...
        for someone sicker...
          in more need... _____

July 6TH

"We need to see with our eyes open and seek out the beautiful and the delightful as it is always present. If only we take the time to look for it. There is something in the human spirit that has been created to do this. It is so obvious to little children. They marvel at the world but sometimes we lose our appreciation for the lives that we have been given as we get older."

—JEANNE SELANDER MILLER
A BREATH AWAY

What I can appreciate again: _____

The best part of my day: _____

Something that made me laugh: _____

Whom did I let "off the hook" today? _____

Someone / Something that brings me joy: _____

Where kindness touched my world today: _____

How I nourished my mind, body or spirit: _____

Number of hours I rested or slept in past 24 hours:
___ Rest ___ Sleep

Prayer/Meditation for the day:
☼ Yes ☼ No

I am grateful for: _____

Today I did this one little thing
    For the earth...
        for a friend or a stranger...
           for someone older or younger...
              for someone sicker...
                in more need... _____

" Our flaws and weaknesses, while often obstacles to our getting work done, are a source of strength as well."

—DAVID BAYLES, TED ORLAND
ART & FEAR: OBSERVATIONS ON THE PERILS (AND REWARDS) OF ARTMAKING

A flaw I have that I can transform into a strength: _____

The best part of my day: _____

Something that made me laugh: _____

Whom did I let "off the hook" today? _____

Someone / Something that brings me joy: _____

Where kindness touched my world today: _____

How I nourished my mind, body or spirit: _____

Number of hours I rested or slept in past 24 hours:
___ Rest   ___ Sleep

Prayer/Meditation for the day:
☼ Yes   ☼ No

I am grateful for: _____

Today I did this one little thing
  For the earth...
    for a friend or a stranger...
      for someone older or younger...
        for someone sicker...
          in more need... _____

July 8TH

"Instead of wanting to know why this had happened, I now began focusing on what I was going to do about it."
—DR. NEIL SPECTOR

Am I focusing on the why or on the action? _____

The best part of my day: _____

Something that made me laugh: _____

Whom did I let "off the hook" today? _____

Someone / Something that brings me joy: _____

Where kindness touched my world today: _____

How I nourished my mind, body or spirit: _____

Number of hours I rested or slept in past 24 hours:
___ Rest ___ Sleep

Prayer/Meditation for the day:
☼ Yes ☼ No

I am grateful for: _____

Today I did this one little thing
    For the earth...
        for a friend or a stranger...
            for someone older or younger...
                for someone sicker...
                    in more need... _____

"Once the storm is over you will not remember how you made it through, how you managed to survive. You won't even be sure, in fact, whether the storm is really over. But one thing is certain, When you come out of the storm you won't be the same person who walked in."
—HARUKI MURAKAMI

How I have changed: _____

The best part of my day: _____

Something that made me laugh: _____

Whom did I let "off the hook" today? _____

Someone / Something that brings me joy: _____

Where kindness touched my world today: _____

How I nourished my mind, body or spirit: _____

Number of hours I rested or slept in past 24 hours:
____ Rest   ____ Sleep

Prayer/Meditation for the day:
☼ Yes   ☼ No

I am grateful for: _____

Today I did this one little thing
　　For the earth...
　　　　for a friend or a stranger...
　　　　　　for someone older or younger...
　　　　　　　　for someone sicker...
　　　　　　　　　　in more need... _____

July 10TH

"Love is so exquisitely elusive. It cannot be bought, cannot be badgered, cannot be hijacked. It is available only in one rare form: as the natural response of a healthy mind and healthy heart."
—EKNATH EASWARAN

When or where I felt loved today: _____

The best part of my day: _____

Something that made me laugh: _____

Whom did I let "off the hook" today? _____

Someone / Something that brings me joy: _____

Where kindness touched my world today: _____

How I nourished my mind, body or spirit: _____

Number of hours I rested or slept in past 24 hours:
___ Rest   ___ Sleep

Prayer/Meditation for the day:
☼ Yes   ☼ No

I am grateful for: _____

Today I did this one little thing
    For the earth...
        for a friend or a stranger...
           for someone older or younger...
               for someone sicker...
                  in more need... _____

Early Month Review

Best part of the past ten days? _____

Number of days I laughed: _____

Goal I want to set for the next 10 days: _____

Person/people who did or
said something to help me heal: _____

Anything else I have noticed
or want to remember/record: _____

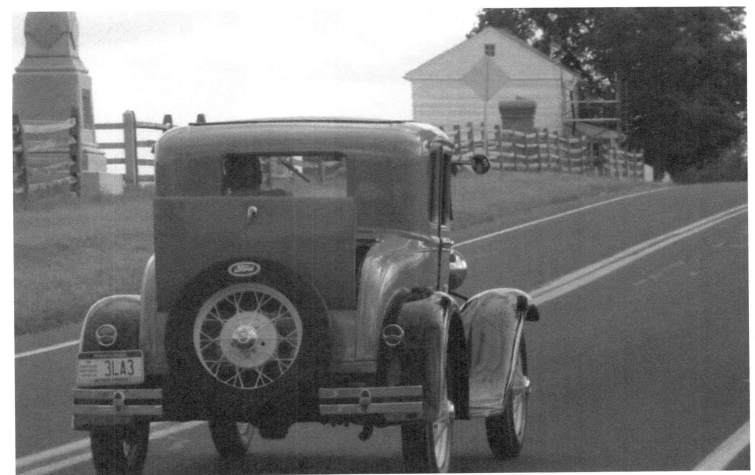

©JOE KELLY

July 11TH

"It is necessary, then, to cultivate the habit of being grateful for every good thing comes to you, and to give thanks continuously. And because all things have contributed to your advancement, you should include all things in your gratitude."
—WALLACE D. WATTLES

I am satisfied with: _____

The best part of my day: _____

Something that made me laugh: _____

Whom did I let "off the hook" today? _____

Someone / Something that brings me joy: _____

Where kindness touched my world today: _____

How I nourished my mind, body or spirit: _____

Number of hours I rested or slept in past 24 hours:
____ Rest   ____ Sleep

Prayer/Meditation for the day:
☼ Yes   ☼ No

I am grateful for: _____

Today I did this one little thing
    For the earth...
        for a friend or a stranger...
           for someone older or younger...
               for someone sicker...
                  in more need... _____

" Whatever you are physically... male or female, strong or weak, ill or healthy—all those things matter less than what your heart contains. If you have the soul of a warrior, you are a warrior. All those other things, they are the glass that contains the lamp, but you are the light inside."
—CASSANDRA CLARE

Who else do I know who is a warrior? _____

The best part of my day: _____

Something that made me laugh: _____

Whom did I let "off the hook" today? _____

Someone / Something that brings me joy: _____

Where kindness touched my world today: _____

How I nourished my mind, body or spirit: _____

Number of hours I rested or slept in past 24 hours:
___ Rest   ___ Sleep

Prayer/Meditation for the day:
☼ Yes   ☼ No

I am grateful for: _____

Today I did this one little thing
    For the earth...
        for a friend or a stranger...
           for someone older or younger...
               for someone sicker...
                  in more need... _____

July 13TH

"Who I truly am is perfect and whole, this body I inhabit has its problems yet it serves me well and I love it and am so very grateful for all of the experiences that it allows me."
—PAULA DAVIS

What parts of me have I accepted? _____

The best part of my day: _____

Something that made me laugh: _____

Whom did I let "off the hook" today? _____

Someone / Something that brings me joy: _____

Where kindness touched my world today: _____

How I nourished my mind, body or spirit: _____

Number of hours I rested or slept in past 24 hours:
____ Rest   ____ Sleep

Prayer/Meditation for the day:
☼ Yes   ☼ No

I am grateful for: _____

Today I did this one little thing
    For the earth...
        for a friend or a stranger...
            for someone older or younger...
                for someone sicker...
                    in more need... _____

"*Courage is the power to let go of the familiar.*"
—DR. RAYMOND I. LINDQUIST

A barrier I broke down: _____

The best part of my day: _____

Something that made me laugh: _____

Whom did I let "off the hook" today? _____

Someone / Something that brings me joy: _____

Where kindness touched my world today: _____

How I nourished my mind, body or spirit: _____

Number of hours I rested or slept in past 24 hours:
___ Rest   ___ Sleep

Prayer/Meditation for the day:
☼ Yes   ☼ No

I am grateful for: _____

Today I did this one little thing
    For the earth...
        for a friend or a stranger...
            for someone older or younger...
                for someone sicker...
                    in more need... _____

July 15TH

" The universe is not required to be in perfect harmony with human ambition. "
—CARL SAGAN

I relinquish: _____

The best part of my day: _____

Something that made me laugh: _____

Whom did I let "off the hook" today? _____

Someone / Something that brings me joy: _____

Where kindness touched my world today: _____

How I nourished my mind, body or spirit: _____

Number of hours I rested or slept in past 24 hours:
____Rest   ____Sleep

Prayer/Meditation for the day:
☼ Yes   ☼ No

I am grateful for: _____

Today I did this one little thing
    For the earth...
        for a friend or a stranger...
            for someone older or younger...
                for someone sicker...
                    in more need... _____

" *You do a lot for other people but what are you doing for yourself?* **"**
—ANGELE RICE

What I did for myself today: _____

The best part of my day: _____

Something that made me laugh: _____

Whom did I let "off the hook" today? _____

Someone / Something that brings me joy: _____

Where kindness touched my world today: _____

How I nourished my mind, body or spirit: _____

Number of hours I rested or slept in past 24 hours:
___Rest   ___Sleep

Prayer/Meditation for the day:
☼ Yes   ☼ No

I am grateful for: _____

Today I did this one little thing
    For the earth...
        for a friend or a stranger...
            for someone older or younger...
                for someone sicker...
                    in more need... _____

July 17TH

"*The way I see it, if you want the rainbow, you gotta put up with the rain.*"
—DOLLY PARTON

The rain and rainbow in my day today: _____

The best part of my day: _____

Something that made me laugh: _____

Whom did I let "off the hook" today? _____

Someone / Something that brings me joy: _____

Where kindness touched my world today: _____

How I nourished my mind, body or spirit: _____

Number of hours I rested or slept in past 24 hours:
___ Rest   ___ Sleep

Prayer/Meditation for the day:
☼ Yes   ☼ No

I am grateful for: _____

Today I did this one little thing
    For the earth...
        for a friend or a stranger...
            for someone older or younger...
                for someone sicker...
                    in more need... _____

" You can't let go of what you haven't held."
—TERRI ST. CLOUD
BONESIGHARTS.COM

Something I held onto for too long: _____

The best part of my day: _____

Something that made me laugh: _____

Whom did I let "off the hook" today? _____

Someone / Something that brings me joy: _____

Where kindness touched my world today: _____

How I nourished my mind, body or spirit: _____

Number of hours I rested or slept in past 24 hours:
___ Rest   ___ Sleep

Prayer/Meditation for the day:
☼ Yes   ☼ No

I am grateful for: _____

Today I did this one little thing
  For the earth...
    for a friend or a stranger...
      for someone older or younger...
        for someone sicker...
          in more need... _____

July 19TH

"Nothing can stop the man with the right mental attitude from achieving his goal; nothing on earth can help the man with the wrong mental attitude."
—THOMAS JEFFERSON

Something I learned: _____

The best part of my day: _____

Something that made me laugh: _____

Whom did I let "off the hook" today? _____

Someone / Something that brings me joy: _____

Where kindness touched my world today: _____

How I nourished my mind, body or spirit: _____

Number of hours I rested or slept in past 24 hours:
___ Rest ___ Sleep

Prayer/Meditation for the day:
☼ Yes ☼ No

I am grateful for: _____

Today I did this one little thing
    For the earth...
        for a friend or a stranger...
           for someone older or younger...
               for someone sicker...
                  in more need... _____

> **❝** *Breath is the bridge which connect life to consciousness, which unites your body to your thoughts.* **❞**
> —THICH NHAT HANH

Did I practice slow, deep breathing today? _____

The best part of my day: _____

Something that made me laugh: _____

Whom did I let "off the hook" today? _____

Someone / Something that brings me joy: _____

Where kindness touched my world today: _____

How I nourished my mind, body or spirit: _____

Number of hours I rested or slept in past 24 hours:
____Rest   ____Sleep

Prayer/Meditation for the day:
☼ Yes   ☼ No

I am grateful for: _____

Today I did this one little thing
      For the earth...
            for a friend or a stranger...
                  for someone older or younger...
                        for someone sicker...
                              in more need... _____

Mid Month
Review

Best part of the past ten days? _____

Number of days I laughed: _____

Goal I want to set for the next 10 days: _____

Person/people who did or
said something to help me heal: _____

Anything else I have noticed
or want to remember/record: _____

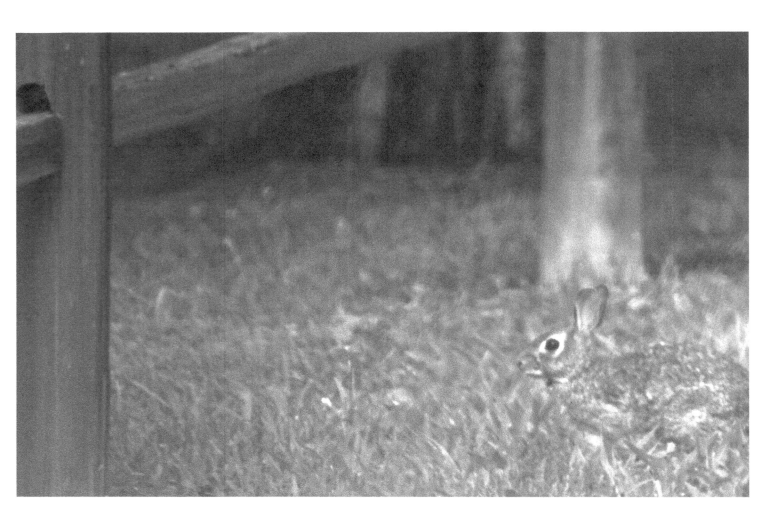

> *"Acceptance opens us to surrendering. Surrendering provides awareness. Awareness provides space for love. Love leads to forgiveness; forgiveness to gratitude; and gratitude to more love. Love heals."*
> —JENNA WRIGHT

What am I opening to? _____

The best part of my day: _____

Something that made me laugh: _____

Whom did I let "off the hook" today? _____

Someone / Something that brings me joy: _____

Where kindness touched my world today: _____

How I nourished my mind, body or spirit: _____

Number of hours I rested or slept in past 24 hours:
____ Rest ____ Sleep

Prayer/Meditation for the day:
☼ Yes ☼ No

I am grateful for: _____

Today I did this one little thing
    For the earth...
        for a friend or a stranger...
            for someone older or younger...
                for someone sicker...
                    in more need... _____

July 22ND

" Through kindness, you can change your fate."
—NGUYEN T. NGUYEN

I showed kindness to _____ today.

The best part of my day: _____

Something that made me laugh: _____

Whom did I let "off the hook" today? _____

Someone / Something that brings me joy: _____

Where kindness touched my world today: _____

How I nourished my mind, body or spirit: _____

Number of hours I rested or slept in past 24 hours:
___ Rest   ___ Sleep

Prayer/Meditation for the day:
☼ Yes   ☼ No

I am grateful for: _____

Today I did this one little thing
   For the earth...
      for a friend or a stranger...
         for someone older or younger...
           for someone sicker...
              in more need... _____

"Revealing is the beginning of Healing. Revelation is the beginning of Transformation."
—TARA SUNSHINE RUAH

Where am I in my Healing and Transformation? _____

The best part of my day: _____

Something that made me laugh: _____

Whom did I let "off the hook" today? _____

Someone / Something that brings me joy: _____

Where kindness touched my world today: _____

How I nourished my mind, body or spirit: _____

Number of hours I rested or slept in past 24 hours:
___ Rest   ___ Sleep

Prayer/Meditation for the day:
☼ Yes   ☼ No

I am grateful for: _____

Today I did this one little thing
    For the earth...
        for a friend or a stranger...
            for someone older or younger...
                for someone sicker...
                    in more need... _____

July 24TH

"Strength does not come from physical capacity. It comes from an indomitable will."
—MAHATMA GANDHI

What or who gave me energy today: _____

The best part of my day: _____

Something that made me laugh: _____

Whom did I let "off the hook" today? _____

Someone / Something that brings me joy: _____

Where kindness touched my world today: _____

How I nourished my mind, body or spirit: _____

Number of hours I rested or slept in past 24 hours:
___ Rest   ___ Sleep

Prayer/Meditation for the day:
☼ Yes   ☼ No

I am grateful for: _____

Today I did this one little thing
    For the earth...
        for a friend or a stranger...
            for someone older or younger...
                for someone sicker...
                    in more need... _____

"*My attitude can affect my recovery from any illness; how I choose to look at the detours in my life can either strengthen me or deplete my energy and recovery.*"
—JANET DECESARE

What I am looking at today that will strengthen me: _____

The best part of my day: _____

Something that made me laugh: _____

Whom did I let "off the hook" today? _____

Someone / Something that brings me joy: _____

Where kindness touched my world today: _____

How I nourished my mind, body or spirit: _____

Number of hours I rested or slept in past 24 hours:
____ Rest   ____ Sleep

Prayer/Meditation for the day:
☼ Yes   ☼ No

I am grateful for: _____

Today I did this one little thing
    For the earth...
        for a friend or a stranger...
            for someone older or younger...
                for someone sicker...
                    in more need... _____

July 26TH

" We need to stop surviving and start living, where we are, with what we have, the best we can. Step by step. "
—ANGELE RICE

Am I living or simply surviving? How? _____

The best part of my day: _____

Something that made me laugh: _____

Whom did I let "off the hook" today? _____

Someone / Something that brings me joy: _____

Where kindness touched my world today: _____

How I nourished my mind, body or spirit: _____

Number of hours I rested or slept in past 24 hours:
___ Rest ___ Sleep

Prayer/Meditation for the day:
☼ Yes ☼ No

I am grateful for: _____

Today I did this one little thing
    For the earth...
        for a friend or a stranger...
           for someone older or younger...
               for someone sicker...
                  in more need... _____

> "*As soon as I became a loner in my own mind, that's when I got what you might call a following. As soon as you stop wanting something you get it. I've found that to be absolutely axiomatic.*"
> —ANDY WARHOL

Did I sit anywhere in silence today? _____

The best part of my day: _____

Something that made me laugh: _____

Whom did I let "off the hook" today? _____

Someone / Something that brings me joy: _____

Where kindness touched my world today: _____

How I nourished my mind, body or spirit: _____

Number of hours I rested or slept in past 24 hours:
___ Rest ___ Sleep

Prayer/Meditation for the day:
☼ Yes ☼ No

I am grateful for: _____

Today I did this one little thing
For the earth...
for a friend or a stranger...
for someone older or younger...
for someone sicker...
in more need... _____

July 28TH

" Our deepest fear is not that we are inadequate. Our deepest fear is that we are powerful beyond measure. It is our light, not our darkness, that most frightens us. "
—MARIANNE WILLIAMSON

A way that I am powerful: _____

The best part of my day: _____

Something that made me laugh: _____

Whom did I let "off the hook" today? _____

Someone / Something that brings me joy: _____

Where kindness touched my world today: _____

How I nourished my mind, body or spirit: _____

Number of hours I rested or slept in past 24 hours:
____ Rest ____ Sleep

Prayer/Meditation for the day:
☼ Yes ☼ No

I am grateful for: _____

Today I did this one little thing
    For the earth...
        for a friend or a stranger...
           for someone older or younger...
               for someone sicker...
                  in more need... _____

" *Every time you are tempted to react in the same old way, ask if you want to be a prisoner of the past or a pioneer of the future.* "

—DEEPAK CHOPRA

What is my choice today? Prisoner or pioneer? _____

The best part of my day: _____

Something that made me laugh: _____

Whom did I let "off the hook" today? _____

Someone / Something that brings me joy: _____

Where kindness touched my world today: _____

How I nourished my mind, body or spirit: _____

Number of hours I rested or slept in past 24 hours:
___ Rest   ___ Sleep

Prayer/Meditation for the day:
☼ Yes   ☼ No

I am grateful for: _____

Today I did this one little thing
    For the earth...
        for a friend or a stranger...
           for someone older or younger...
              for someone sicker...
                in more need... _____

July 30TH

" Colors are the smiles of nature. **"**
—LEIGH HUNT

What color I saw today that resonated: _____

The best part of my day: _____

Something that made me laugh: _____

Whom did I let "off the hook" today? _____

Someone / Something that brings me joy: _____

Where kindness touched my world today: _____

How I nourished my mind, body or spirit: _____

Number of hours I rested or slept in past 24 hours:
___Rest   ___Sleep

Prayer/Meditation for the day:
☀ Yes   ☀ No

I am grateful for: _____

Today I did this one little thing
   For the earth...
      for a friend or a stranger...
         for someone older or younger...
           for someone sicker...
              in more need... _____

> " *Being in the quiet allows me to be aware. Being in the quiet allows me to think my thoughts, and to express them in my own stories.* "
> —SHARON RAINEY

Did I have some quiet time today? _____

The best part of my day: _____

Something that made me laugh: _____

Whom did I let "off the hook" today? _____

Someone / Something that brings me joy: _____

Where kindness touched my world today: _____

How I nourished my mind, body or spirit: _____

Number of hours I rested or slept in past 24 hours:
___ Rest   ___ Sleep

Prayer/Meditation for the day:
☼ Yes   ☼ No

I am grateful for: _____

Today I did this one little thing
    For the earth...
        for a friend or a stranger...
            for someone older or younger...
                for someone sicker...
                    in more need... _____

10 Day Overview

Best part of the past ten days? _____

Number of days I laughed: _____

Goal I want to set for the next 10 days: _____

Person/people who did or
said something to help me heal: _____

Anything else I have noticed
or want to remember/record: _____

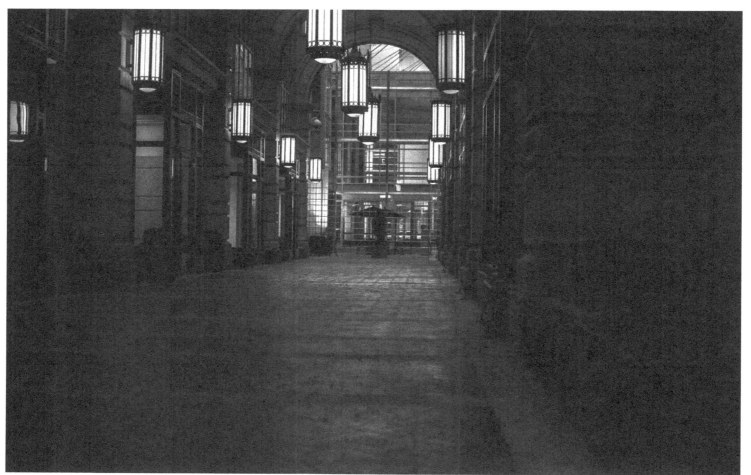

©STEPHEN RAINEY

> *"Not everything that is faced can be changed,*
> *but nothing can be changed until it is faced."*
> —LUCILLE BALL

Something I faced today: _____

The best part of my day: _____

Something that made me laugh: _____

Whom did I let "off the hook" today? _____

Someone / Something that brings me joy: _____

Where kindness touched my world today: _____

How I nourished my mind, body or spirit: _____

Number of hours I rested or slept in past 24 hours:
___Rest   ___Sleep

Prayer/Meditation for the day:
☼ Yes   ☼ No

I am grateful for: _____

Today I did this one little thing
　　For the earth...
　　　　for a friend or a stranger...
　　　　　　for someone older or younger...
　　　　　　　　for someone sicker...
　　　　　　　　　　in more need... _____

August 2ND

"Smell is a potent wizard that transports you across thousands of miles and all the years you have lived."
—HELEN KELLER

Favorite scent I smelled today: _____

The best part of my day: _____

Something that made me laugh: _____

Whom did I let "off the hook" today? _____

Someone / Something that brings me joy: _____

Where kindness touched my world today: _____

How I nourished my mind, body or spirit: _____

Number of hours I rested or slept in past 24 hours:
____ Rest   ____ Sleep

Prayer/Meditation for the day:
☼ Yes   ☼ No

I am grateful for: _____

Today I did this one little thing
    For the earth...
        for a friend or a stranger...
            for someone older or younger...
                for someone sicker...
                    in more need... _____

*"Don't run away from a challenge. Instead run toward it, because
the only way to escape fear is to trample it beneath your feet."*
—NADIA COMANECI

How I faced a fear: _____

The best part of my day: _____

Something that made me laugh: _____

Whom did I let "off the hook" today? _____

Someone / Something that brings me joy: _____

Where kindness touched my world today: _____

How I nourished my mind, body or spirit: _____

Number of hours I rested or slept in past 24 hours:
___ Rest   ___ Sleep

Prayer/Meditation for the day:
☼ Yes   ☼ No

I am grateful for: _____

Today I did this one little thing
    For the earth...
        for a friend or a stranger...
           for someone older or younger...
             for someone sicker...
                in more need... _____

August 4TH

"Living your purpose is your most powerful and successful life accomplishment. It gives your life meaning, fulfillment, joy, peace, and happiness that you cannot get from external sources. You shift from being self-conscious to self-confident. The light that shines within you will align with the universe, and everything you need will be supplied."

—CATHY HOLLOWAY HILL

INSPIREMETODAY.COM/BRILLIANCE/HOW-DO-YOU-DEFINE-SUCCESS

Favorite scent I smelled today: _____

The best part of my day: _____

Something that made me laugh: _____

Whom did I let "off the hook" today? _____

Someone / Something that brings me joy: _____

Where kindness touched my world today: _____

How I nourished my mind, body or spirit: _____

Number of hours I rested or slept in past 24 hours:
____ Rest   ____ Sleep

Prayer/Meditation for the day:
☼ Yes   ☼ No

I am grateful for: _____

Today I did this one little thing
　　For the earth...
　　　　for a friend or a stranger...
　　　　　　for someone older or younger...
　　　　　　　　for someone sicker...
　　　　　　　　　　in more need... _____

" Happiness is something that comes into our lives
through doors we don't even remember leaving open."
—ROSE LANE

Do I want to be right or do I want to be happy? _____

The best part of my day: _____

Something that made me laugh: _____

Whom did I let "off the hook" today? _____

Someone / Something that brings me joy: _____

Where kindness touched my world today: _____

How I nourished my mind, body or spirit: _____

Number of hours I rested or slept in past 24 hours:
___ Rest   ___ Sleep

Prayer/Meditation for the day:
☼ Yes   ☼ No

I am grateful for: _____

Today I did this one little thing
    For the earth...
        for a friend or a stranger...
            for someone older or younger...
                for someone sicker...
                    in more need... _____

August 6TH

" The truth is that our finest moments are most likely to occur when we are feeling deeply uncomfortable, unhappy, or unfulfilled. For it is only in such moments, propelled by our discomfort, that we are likely to step out of our ruts and start searching for different ways or truer answers. "

—ANONYMOUS

How did I step out of a rut: _____

The best part of my day: _____

Something that made me laugh: _____

Whom did I let "off the hook" today? _____

Someone / Something that brings me joy: _____

Where kindness touched my world today: _____

How I nourished my mind, body or spirit: _____

Number of hours I rested or slept in past 24 hours:
___ Rest ___ Sleep

Prayer/Meditation for the day:
☼ Yes ☼ No

I am grateful for: _____

Today I did this one little thing
    For the earth...
        for a friend or a stranger...
           for someone older or younger...
               for someone sicker...
                  in more need... _____

> " *Words, once received by the mind, become food for the soul. Let us be mindful to speak nutritiously.* "
> —JENNA WRIGHT

Am I feeding my soul in a healthy way? _____

The best part of my day: _____

Something that made me laugh: _____

Whom did I let "off the hook" today? _____

Someone / Something that brings me joy: _____

Where kindness touched my world today: _____

How I nourished my mind, body or spirit: _____

Number of hours I rested or slept in past 24 hours:
____ Rest   ____ Sleep

Prayer/Meditation for the day:
☼ Yes   ☼ No

I am grateful for: _____

Today I did this one little thing
    For the earth...
        for a friend or a stranger...
            for someone older or younger...
                for someone sicker...
                    in more need... _____

August 8TH

" *To be happy, we must not be too concerned with others.* "
—ALBERT CAMUS

Am I improving on setting boundaries with others? _____

The best part of my day: _____

Something that made me laugh: _____

Whom did I let "off the hook" today? _____

Someone / Something that brings me joy: _____

Where kindness touched my world today: _____

How I nourished my mind, body or spirit: _____

Number of hours I rested or slept in past 24 hours:
___ Rest   ___ Sleep

Prayer/Meditation for the day:
☼ Yes   ☼ No

I am grateful for: _____

Today I did this one little thing
     For the earth...
          for a friend or a stranger...
               for someone older or younger...
                    for someone sicker...
                         in more need... _____

> " *There is darkness in the world, but it is merely an absence of light. All the darkness in the world cannot dispel even the smallest candle flame. We need only accustom ourselves to the dim vision, and then the blessing of light will grow.* "
> —AUNG SAN SUU KYI
> *FREEDOM FROM FEAR: AND OTHER WRITINGS*

A fear that I am working to conquer: _____

The best part of my day: _____

Something that made me laugh: _____

Whom did I let "off the hook" today? _____

Someone / Something that brings me joy: _____

Where kindness touched my world today: _____

How I nourished my mind, body or spirit: _____

Number of hours I rested or slept in past 24 hours:
___ Rest ___ Sleep

Prayer/Meditation for the day:
☼ Yes ☼ No

I am grateful for: _____

Today I did this one little thing
For the earth...
for a friend or a stranger...
for someone older or younger...
for someone sicker...
in more need... _____

August 10TH

> " *The strongest people are not those who show strength in front of us, but those who win battles we know nothing about.* "
> —ROBIN SEABROOK

Another strong person I know: _____

The best part of my day: _____

Something that made me laugh: _____

Whom did I let "off the hook" today? _____

Someone / Something that brings me joy: _____

Where kindness touched my world today: _____

How I nourished my mind, body or spirit: _____

Number of hours I rested or slept in past 24 hours:
___ Rest   ___ Sleep

Prayer/Meditation for the day:
☼ Yes   ☼ No

I am grateful for: _____

Today I did this one little thing
    For the earth...
        for a friend or a stranger...
            for someone older or younger...
                for someone sicker...
                    in more need... _____

Early Month Review

Best part of the past ten days? _____

Number of days I laughed: _____

Goal I want to set for the next 10 days: _____

Person/people who did or
said something to help me heal: _____

Anything else I have noticed
or want to remember/record: _____

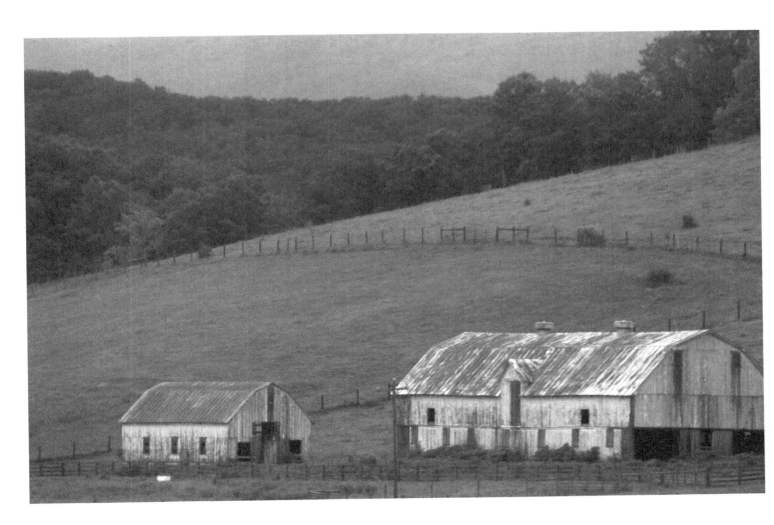

August 11TH

> *"I have tried to make compassion a life habit. I think of it as practicing magic."*
> —MARY MIDKIFF

Something I am ready to celebrate or celebrated: _____

The best part of my day: _____

Something that made me laugh: _____

Whom did I let "off the hook" today? _____

Someone / Something that brings me joy: _____

Where kindness touched my world today: _____

How I nourished my mind, body or spirit: _____

Number of hours I rested or slept in past 24 hours:
___ Rest   ___ Sleep

Prayer/Meditation for the day:
☼ Yes   ☼ No

I am grateful for: _____

Today I did this one little thing
    For the earth...
        for a friend or a stranger...
            for someone older or younger...
               for someone sicker...
                  in more need... _____

August 12TH

> *"Healing is a conscious choice I make each day; one that comes with great hardship yet brings the reward worth the struggle, which is to wake again the next dawn in gratitude despite all else."*
> —KARA THOMMEN

What conscious choices am I making
today to enable an attitude of gratitude? _____

The best part of my day: _____

Something that made me laugh: _____

Whom did I let "off the hook" today? _____

Someone / Something that brings me joy: _____

Where kindness touched my world today: _____

How I nourished my mind, body or spirit: _____

Number of hours I rested or slept in past 24 hours:
___ Rest   ___ Sleep

Prayer/Meditation for the day:
☼ Yes   ☼ No

I am grateful for: _____

Today I did this one little thing
    For the earth...
        for a friend or a stranger...
           for someone older or younger...
              for someone sicker...
                in more need... _____

August 13TH

" My humanity is caught up, is inextricably bound up, with others. We belong in a bundle of life. A person is a person through other people. "

—DESMOND TUTU
NO FUTURE WITHOUT FORGIVENESS

Something I am ready to celebrate or celebrated: _____

The best part of my day: _____

Something that made me laugh: _____

Whom did I let "off the hook" today? _____

Someone / Something that brings me joy: _____

Where kindness touched my world today: _____

How I nourished my mind, body or spirit: _____

Number of hours I rested or slept in past 24 hours:
___ Rest   ___ Sleep

Prayer/Meditation for the day:
☼ Yes   ☼ No

I am grateful for: _____

Today I did this one little thing
    For the earth...
        for a friend or a stranger...
            for someone older or younger...
                for someone sicker...
                    in more need... _____

*" We have no right to ask when sorrow comes, Why did this happen to me? unless
we ask the same question for every moment of happiness that comes our way."*
—ANONYMOUS

I want to add: _____

The best part of my day: _____

Something that made me laugh: _____

Whom did I let "off the hook" today? _____

Someone / Something that brings me joy: _____

Where kindness touched my world today: _____

How I nourished my mind, body or spirit: _____

Number of hours I rested or slept in past 24 hours:
___ Rest   ___ Sleep

Prayer/Meditation for the day:
☼ Yes   ☼ No

I am grateful for: _____

Today I did this one little thing
     For the earth...
          for a friend or a stranger...
               for someone older or younger...
                    for someone sicker...
                         in more need... _____

August 15TH

" Don't compare your journey to someone else's; it devalues their story and yours. "
—ANGELE RICE

Something unique about me: _____

The best part of my day: _____

Something that made me laugh: _____

Whom did I let "off the hook" today? _____

Someone / Something that brings me joy: _____

Where kindness touched my world today: _____

How I nourished my mind, body or spirit: _____

Number of hours I rested or slept in past 24 hours:
___Rest   ___Sleep

Prayer/Meditation for the day:
☼ Yes   ☼ No

I am grateful for: _____

Today I did this one little thing
For the earth...
for a friend or a stranger...
for someone older or younger...
for someone sicker...
in more need... _____

August 16TH

"*Action may not always bring happiness; but there is no happiness without action.*"
—BENJAMIN DISRAELI

One small detail I addressed
that made my life easier: _____

The best part of my day: _____

Something that made me laugh: _____

Whom did I let "off the hook" today? _____

Someone / Something that brings me joy: _____

Where kindness touched my world today: _____

How I nourished my mind, body or spirit: _____

Number of hours I rested or slept in past 24 hours:
____ Rest   ____ Sleep

Prayer/Meditation for the day:
☼ Yes   ☼ No

I am grateful for: _____

Today I did this one little thing
    For the earth...
        for a friend or a stranger...
            for someone older or younger...
                for someone sicker...
                    in more need... _____

August 17TH

"Some fears can be conquered... Others have a way of coming back around. Sometimes at the moment you least expect. Often with the very worst possible timing. Fear makes it hard to think. And when you can't think, it's hard to figure out your choices. When you can't see all your options, all you can do is react."

—INGRID LAW
SCUMBLE

I am no longer afraid of: _____

The best part of my day: _____

Something that made me laugh: _____

Whom did I let "off the hook" today? _____

Someone / Something that brings me joy: _____

Where kindness touched my world today: _____

How I nourished my mind, body or spirit: _____

Number of hours I rested or slept in past 24 hours:
____Rest   ____Sleep

Prayer/Meditation for the day:
☼ Yes   ☼ No

I am grateful for: _____

Today I did this one little thing
    For the earth...
        for a friend or a stranger...
            for someone older or younger...
                for someone sicker...
                    in more need... _____

" *I believe the direction of our lives is more important than the speed at which we travel.* "
—HARRIET GOLDHOR LEARNER

I believe: _____

The best part of my day: _____

Something that made me laugh: _____

Whom did I let "off the hook" today? _____

Someone / Something that brings me joy: _____

Where kindness touched my world today: _____

How I nourished my mind, body or spirit: _____

Number of hours I rested or slept in past 24 hours:
___ Rest ___ Sleep

Prayer/Meditation for the day:
☼ Yes ☼ No

I am grateful for: _____

Today I did this one little thing
 For the earth...
  for a friend or a stranger...
   for someone older or younger...
    for someone sicker...
     in more need... _____

August 19TH

> *"And the fist became the open hand. She refused to beat herself any longer. Speaking words of kindness, she gently touched her hair, looked into her own eyes and took the first step towards love."*
>
> —TERRI ST. CLOUD
> BONESIGHARTS.COM

A time when I chose love over pain: _____

The best part of my day: _____

Something that made me laugh: _____

Whom did I let "off the hook" today? _____

Someone / Something that brings me joy: _____

Where kindness touched my world today: _____

How I nourished my mind, body or spirit: _____

Number of hours I rested or slept in past 24 hours:
___ Rest   ___ Sleep

Prayer/Meditation for the day:
☼ Yes   ☼ No

I am grateful for: _____

Today I did this one little thing
    For the earth...
        for a friend or a stranger...
            for someone older or younger...
                for someone sicker...
                    in more need... _____

❝ *Beauty is not in the face; beauty is a light in the heart.* ❞
—KHALIL GIBRAN

Do I see light in my own heart? In others' hearts? _____

The best part of my day: _____

Something that made me laugh: _____

Whom did I let "off the hook" today? _____

Someone / Something that brings me joy: _____

Where kindness touched my world today: _____

How I nourished my mind, body or spirit: _____

Number of hours I rested or slept in past 24 hours:
___ Rest ___ Sleep

Prayer/Meditation for the day:
☼ Yes ☼ No

I am grateful for: _____

Today I did this one little thing
    For the earth...
        for a friend or a stranger...
           for someone older or younger...
              for someone sicker...
                in more need... _____

Mid Month
Review

Best part of the past ten days? _____

Number of days I laughed: _____

Goal I want to set for the next 10 days: _____

Person/people who did or
said something to help me heal: _____

Anything else I have noticed
or want to remember/record: _____

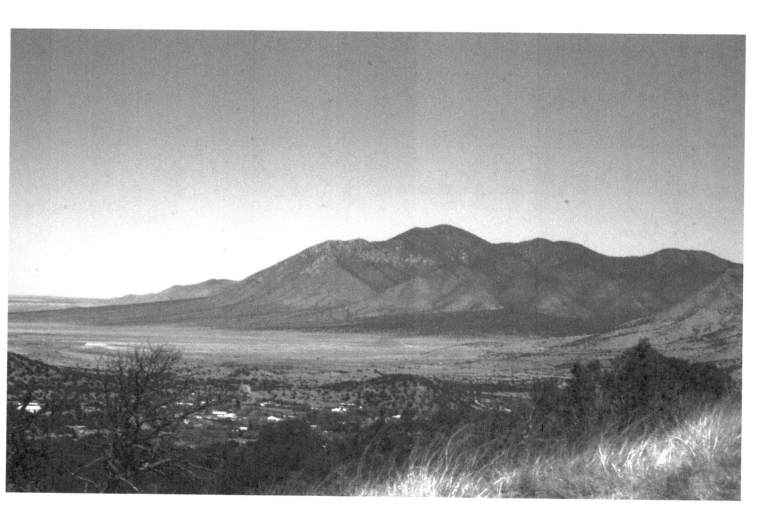

"*Excellence is not a singular act, but a habit. You are what you repeatedly do.*"
—ARISTOTLE

If I am what I repeatedly do, what am I? What do I want to be? How can I transform this desire into a habit? _____

The best part of my day: _____

Something that made me laugh: _____

Whom did I let "off the hook" today? _____

Someone / Something that brings me joy: _____

Where kindness touched my world today: _____

How I nourished my mind, body or spirit: _____

Number of hours I rested or slept in past 24 hours:
____ Rest ____ Sleep

Prayer/Meditation for the day:
☼ Yes ☼ No

I am grateful for: _____

Today I did this one little thing
    For the earth...
        for a friend or a stranger...
           for someone older or younger...
              for someone sicker...
                in more need... _____

August 22ND

"Happiness can exist only in acceptance."
—GEORGE ORWELL

What am I accepting of today? _____

The best part of my day: _____

Something that made me laugh: _____

Whom did I let "off the hook" today? _____

Someone / Something that brings me joy: _____

Where kindness touched my world today: _____

How I nourished my mind, body or spirit: _____

Number of hours I rested or slept in past 24 hours:
___ Rest ___ Sleep

Prayer/Meditation for the day:
☼ Yes   ☼ No

I am grateful for: _____

Today I did this one little thing
    For the earth...
        for a friend or a stranger...
            for someone older or younger...
                for someone sicker...
                    in more need... _____

August 23RD

"It's just about impossible to make Positive changes in a Negative enviroment. And Sometimes that negative enviroment is simply the thoughts you are surrounding yourself with. Don't corner yourself in, but if you do, let others who love you pull you on out."
—ALISA TURNER

What I can do today to make my
'environment' more positive: _____

The best part of my day: _____

Something that made me laugh: _____

Whom did I let "off the hook" today? _____

Someone / Something that brings me joy: _____

Where kindness touched my world today: _____

How I nourished my mind, body or spirit: _____

Number of hours I rested or slept in past 24 hours:
___ Rest ___ Sleep

Prayer/Meditation for the day:
☼ Yes ☼ No

I am grateful for: _____

Today I did this one little thing
    For the earth...
        for a friend or a stranger...
            for someone older or younger...
                for someone sicker...
                    in more need... _____

August 24TH

> **"** *Being deeply loved by someone gives you strength,*
> *while loving someone deeply gives you courage.* **"**
> —LOU TZU

I love: _____

The best part of my day: _____

Something that made me laugh: _____

Whom did I let "off the hook" today? _____

Someone / Something that brings me joy: _____

Where kindness touched my world today: _____

How I nourished my mind, body or spirit: _____

Number of hours I rested or slept in past 24 hours:
___ Rest   ___ Sleep

Prayer/Meditation for the day:
☼ Yes   ☼ No

I am grateful for: _____

Today I did this one little thing
   For the earth...
      for a friend or a stranger...
         for someone older or younger...
            for someone sicker...
               in more need... _____

August 25TH

"Be gracious in accepting care and assistance from those that love you. Never let the pain isolate you so it becomes too difficult to give and accept that love and care. It is those gifts of love that will carry you through the hardest moments."
—ALYSSA KNAPP

What gifts did I accept today? _____

The best part of my day: _____

Something that made me laugh: _____

Whom did I let "off the hook" today? _____

Someone / Something that brings me joy: _____

Where kindness touched my world today: _____

How I nourished my mind, body or spirit: _____

Number of hours I rested or slept in past 24 hours:
____ Rest ____ Sleep

Prayer/Meditation for the day:
☼ Yes ☼ No

I am grateful for: _____

Today I did this one little thing
    For the earth...
        for a friend or a stranger...
            for someone older or younger...
                for someone sicker...
                    in more need... _____

August 26TH

> *"It is gratefulness which makes the soul great."*
> —ABRAHAM JOSHUA HESCHEL

I am grateful for: _____

The best part of my day: _____

Something that made me laugh: _____

Whom did I let "off the hook" today? _____

Someone / Something that brings me joy: _____

Where kindness touched my world today: _____

How I nourished my mind, body or spirit: _____

Number of hours I rested or slept in past 24 hours:
___ Rest   ___ Sleep

Prayer/Meditation for the day:
☼ Yes   ☼ No

I am grateful for: _____

Today I did this one little thing
　　For the earth...
　　　　for a friend or a stranger...
　　　　　　for someone older or younger...
　　　　　　　　for someone sicker...
　　　　　　　　　　in more need... _____

" *Grace doesn't depend on suffering to exist, but where there is suffering you will find grace in many facets and colors.* "
—WM. PAUL YOUNG

Of all of its facets and colors, what
form does grace take in my life? _____

The best part of my day: _____

Something that made me laugh: _____

Whom did I let "off the hook" today? _____

Someone / Something that brings me joy: _____

Where kindness touched my world today: _____

How I nourished my mind, body or spirit: _____

Number of hours I rested or slept in past 24 hours:
___ Rest   ___ Sleep

Prayer/Meditation for the day:
☼ Yes   ☼ No

I am grateful for: _____

Today I did this one little thing
    For the earth...
        for a friend or a stranger...
            for someone older or younger...
                for someone sicker...
                    in more need... _____

August 28TH

> "*All illnesses are physical, mental, and spiritual, and the highest
> levels of recovery are the consequence of simultaneously addressing
> all three levels and seeing them as being of equal importance.*"
> —DAVID HAWKINS, MD
> *HEALING AND RECOVERY*

Something I did today that I have never done
before or that I did differently than usual: _____

The best part of my day: _____

Something that made me laugh: _____

Whom did I let "off the hook" today? _____

Someone / Something that brings me joy: _____

Where kindness touched my world today: _____

How I nourished my mind, body or spirit: _____

Number of hours I rested or slept in past 24 hours:
____ Rest   ____ Sleep

Prayer/Meditation for the day:
☼ Yes   ☼ No

I am grateful for: _____

Today I did this one little thing
    For the earth...
        for a friend or a stranger...
            for someone older or younger...
                for someone sicker...
                    in more need... _____

"*One is loved because one is loved. No reason is needed for loving.*"
—PAULO COELHO

Someone I love just because: _____

The best part of my day: _____

Something that made me laugh: _____

Whom did I let "off the hook" today? _____

Someone / Something that brings me joy: _____

Where kindness touched my world today: _____

How I nourished my mind, body or spirit: _____

Number of hours I rested or slept in past 24 hours:
___Rest   ___Sleep

Prayer/Meditation for the day:
☼ Yes   ☼ No

I am grateful for: _____

Today I did this one little thing
    For the earth...
        for a friend or a stranger...
            for someone older or younger...
                for someone sicker...
                    in more need... _____

August 30TH

> **"** *Some beautiful things are more impressive when left imperfect than when too highly finished.* **"**
> —FRANÇOIS DE LA ROCHEFOUCAULD

Something I savored: _____

The best part of my day: _____

Something that made me laugh: _____

Whom did I let "off the hook" today? _____

Someone / Something that brings me joy: _____

Where kindness touched my world today: _____

How I nourished my mind, body or spirit: _____

Number of hours I rested or slept in past 24 hours:
____Rest   ____Sleep

Prayer/Meditation for the day:
☼ Yes   ☼ No

I am grateful for: _____

Today I did this one little thing
    For the earth...
        for a friend or a stranger...
            for someone older or younger...
                for someone sicker...
                    in more need... _____

"*Sometimes you gotta create what you want to be a part of.***"**
—GERI WEITZMAN

Something I helped create: _____

The best part of my day: _____

Something that made me laugh: _____

Whom did I let "off the hook" today? _____

Someone / Something that brings me joy: _____

Where kindness touched my world today: _____

How I nourished my mind, body or spirit: _____

Number of hours I rested or slept in past 24 hours:
___ Rest   ___ Sleep

Prayer/Meditation for the day:
☼ Yes   ☼ No

I am grateful for: _____

Today I did this one little thing
  For the earth...
    for a friend or a stranger...
      for someone older or younger...
        for someone sicker...
          in more need... _____

End of Month Review

Best part of the past ten days? _____

Number of days I laughed: _____

Goal I want to set for the next 10 days: _____

Person/people who did or
said something to help me heal: _____

Anything else I have noticed
or want to remember/record: _____

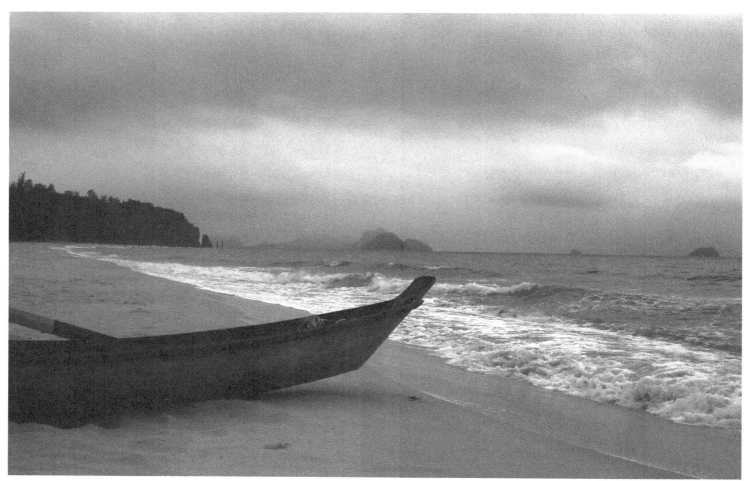

©JOE KELLY

September 1ˢᵀ

" Your work is to discover your work and then give your heart to it. "
—BUDDHA

A creative talent I have: _____

The best part of my day: _____

Something that made me laugh: _____

Whom did I let "off the hook" today? _____

Someone / Something that brings me joy: _____

Where kindness touched my world today: _____

How I nourished my mind, body or spirit: _____

Number of hours I rested or slept in past 24 hours:
____Rest   ____Sleep

Prayer/Meditation for the day:
☼ Yes   ☼ No

I am grateful for: _____

Today I did this one little thing
    For the earth...
        for a friend or a stranger...
            for someone older or younger...
                for someone sicker...
                    in more need... _____

September 2ND

*" Real courage is when you know you're licked before you begin,
but you begin anyway and see it through no matter what. "*
—HARPER LEE

Something that took courage: _____

The best part of my day: _____

Something that made me laugh: _____

Whom did I let "off the hook" today? _____

Someone / Something that brings me joy: _____

Where kindness touched my world today: _____

How I nourished my mind, body or spirit: _____

Number of hours I rested or slept in past 24 hours:
___ Rest ___ Sleep

Prayer/Meditation for the day:
☼ Yes   ☼ No

I am grateful for: _____

Today I did this one little thing
    For the earth...
        for a friend or a stranger...
           for someone older or younger...
              for someone sicker...
                in more need... _____

September 3RD

> " *There will never been enough time given over to the glory of nature simply being itself in everyday ways, and to the beauty and poignancy of time passing.* "
> —ELIZABETH BERG
> FACEBOOK 10/14/16

A creative talent I have: _____

The best part of my day: _____

Something that made me laugh: _____

Whom did I let "off the hook" today? _____

Someone / Something that brings me joy: _____

Where kindness touched my world today: _____

How I nourished my mind, body or spirit: _____

Number of hours I rested or slept in past 24 hours:
___ Rest   ___ Sleep

Prayer/Meditation for the day:
☼ Yes   ☼ No

I am grateful for: _____

Today I did this one little thing
    For the earth...
        for a friend or a stranger...
            for someone older or younger...
                for someone sicker...
                    in more need... _____

September 4TH

" Nothing ever turns out how you plan it to. Sometimes it turns out better. "
—ROBIN SHIRLEY
WWW.ROBINSHIRLEY.COM

Something that turned out better
than I had planned for it to: _____

The best part of my day: _____

Something that made me laugh: _____

Whom did I let "off the hook" today? _____

Someone / Something that brings me joy: _____

Where kindness touched my world today: _____

How I nourished my mind, body or spirit: _____

Number of hours I rested or slept in past 24 hours:
____ Rest   ____ Sleep

Prayer/Meditation for the day:
☼ Yes   ☼ No

I am grateful for: _____

Today I did this one little thing
    For the earth...
        for a friend or a stranger...
           for someone older or younger...
               for someone sicker...
                  in more need... _____

September 5TH

"If you're going through hell, keep going."
—WINSTON CHURCHILL

I am proud of: _____

The best part of my day: _____

Something that made me laugh: _____

Whom did I let "off the hook" today? _____

Someone / Something that brings me joy: _____

Where kindness touched my world today: _____

How I nourished my mind, body or spirit: _____

Number of hours I rested or slept in past 24 hours:
___ Rest   ___ Sleep

Prayer/Meditation for the day:
☀ Yes   ☀ No

I am grateful for: _____

Today I did this one little thing
    For the earth...
        for a friend or a stranger...
            for someone older or younger...
                for someone sicker...
                    in more need... _____

September 6TH

" Defeat is not the worst of failures. Not to have tried is the true failure. "
—GEORGE EDWARD WOODBERRY

A failure that eventually led to something good: _____

The best part of my day: _____

Something that made me laugh: _____

Whom did I let "off the hook" today? _____

Someone / Something that brings me joy: _____

Where kindness touched my world today: _____

How I nourished my mind, body or spirit: _____

Number of hours I rested or slept in past 24 hours:
___ Rest   ___ Sleep

Prayer/Meditation for the day:
☼ Yes   ☼ No

I am grateful for: _____

Today I did this one little thing
    For the earth...
        for a friend or a stranger...
           for someone older or younger...
               for someone sicker...
                  in more need... _____

September 7th

> " *Has a man gained anything who has received a hundred favors and rendered none? He is great who confers the most benefits—* "
> —RALPH WALDO EMERSON

Today I helped: _____

The best part of my day: _____

Something that made me laugh: _____

Whom did I let "off the hook" today? _____

Someone / Something that brings me joy: _____

Where kindness touched my world today: _____

How I nourished my mind, body or spirit: _____

Number of hours I rested or slept in past 24 hours:
____ Rest   ____ Sleep

Prayer/Meditation for the day:
☼ Yes   ☼ No

I am grateful for: _____

Today I did this one little thing
    For the earth...
        for a friend or a stranger...
           for someone older or younger...
               for someone sicker...
                  in more need... _____

September 8TH

"I discovered I always have choices and sometimes it's only a choice of attitude."
—JUDITH KNOWLTON

I choose to: _____

The best part of my day: _____

Something that made me laugh: _____

Whom did I let "off the hook" today? _____

Someone / Something that brings me joy: _____

Where kindness touched my world today: _____

How I nourished my mind, body or spirit: _____

Number of hours I rested or slept in past 24 hours:
___ Rest ___ Sleep

Prayer/Meditation for the day:
☼ Yes ☼ No

I am grateful for: _____

Today I did this one little thing
    For the earth...
        for a friend or a stranger...
            for someone older or younger...
                for someone sicker...
                    in more need... _____

September 9TH

" Keep away from people who try to belittle your ambitions. Small people always do that, but the really great make you feel that you too can become great. "
—MARK TWAIN

Who makes me feel really great? _____

The best part of my day: _____

Something that made me laugh: _____

Whom did I let "off the hook" today? _____

Someone / Something that brings me joy: _____

Where kindness touched my world today: _____

How I nourished my mind, body or spirit: _____

Number of hours I rested or slept in past 24 hours:
___ Rest ___ Sleep

Prayer/Meditation for the day:
☼ Yes ☼ No

I am grateful for: _____

Today I did this one little thing
   For the earth...
      for a friend or a stranger...
         for someone older or younger...
            for someone sicker...
               in more need... _____

September 10TH

"Consult not your fears but your hopes and dreams. Think not about your frustrations but about your unfulfilled potential. Concern yourself not with what you tried and failed in, but what is still possible for you to do."

—POPE PAUL XXIII

It is still possible for me to: _____

The best part of my day: _____

Something that made me laugh: _____

Whom did I let "off the hook" today? _____

Someone / Something that brings me joy: _____

Where kindness touched my world today: _____

How I nourished my mind, body or spirit: _____

Number of hours I rested or slept in past 24 hours:
___ Rest   ___ Sleep

Prayer/Meditation for the day:
☼ Yes   ☼ No

I am grateful for: _____

Today I did this one little thing
    For the earth...
        for a friend or a stranger...
           for someone older or younger...
              for someone sicker...
                in more need... _____

Early Month Review

Best part of the past ten days? _____

Number of days I laughed: _____

Goal I want to set for the next 10 days: _____

Person/people who did or
said something to help me heal: _____

Anything else I have noticed
or want to remember/record: _____

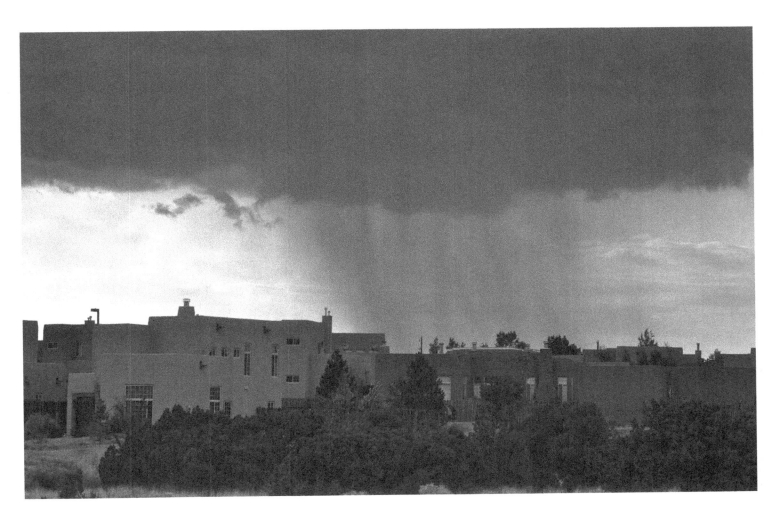

September 11TH

> **"***She's a good person to hug, because her body fills up all the empty spaces.***"**
> —ANITA SHREVE
> *BODY SURFING: A NOVEL*

The last person I hugged: _____

The best part of my day: _____

Something that made me laugh: _____

Whom did I let "off the hook" today? _____

Someone / Something that brings me joy: _____

Where kindness touched my world today: _____

How I nourished my mind, body or spirit: _____

Number of hours I rested or slept in past 24 hours:
___ Rest   ___ Sleep

Prayer/Meditation for the day:
☼ Yes   ☼ No

I am grateful for: _____

Today I did this one little thing
    For the earth...
        for a friend or a stranger...
           for someone older or younger...
               for someone sicker...
                  in more need... _____

September 12TH

"As soon as you trust yourself you will know how to live."
—JOHANN WOLFGANG VON GOETHE

I trust: _____

The best part of my day: _____

Something that made me laugh: _____

Whom did I let "off the hook" today? _____

Someone / Something that brings me joy: _____

Where kindness touched my world today: _____

How I nourished my mind, body or spirit: _____

Number of hours I rested or slept in past 24 hours:
___ Rest   ___ Sleep

Prayer/Meditation for the day:
☼ Yes   ☼ No

I am grateful for: _____

Today I did this one little thing
    For the earth...
        for a friend or a stranger...
            for someone older or younger...
                for someone sicker...
                    in more need... _____

September 13TH

> "*Humbleness, forgiveness, clarity and love are the dynamics of freedom. They are the foundations of authentic power.*"
> —GARY ZUKAV

How I have gained freedom: _____

The best part of my day: _____

Something that made me laugh: _____

Whom did I let "off the hook" today? _____

Someone / Something that brings me joy: _____

Where kindness touched my world today: _____

How I nourished my mind, body or spirit: _____

Number of hours I rested or slept in past 24 hours:
___Rest   ___Sleep

Prayer/Meditation for the day:
☼ Yes   ☼ No

I am grateful for: _____

Today I did this one little thing
    For the earth...
        for a friend or a stranger...
            for someone older or younger...
                for someone sicker...
                    in more need... _____

September 14TH

"It's ok to take baby steps as long as you go in the direction of trust. The next time you're inspired to do something, honor it. That's the Divine talking."
—DR. JOE VITALE
THE MIRACLES MANUAL: THE SECRET COACHING SESSIONS VOLUME 2

What I did today to show my
trust in the healing process: _____

The best part of my day: _____

Something that made me laugh: _____

Whom did I let "off the hook" today? _____

Someone / Something that brings me joy: _____

Where kindness touched my world today: _____

How I nourished my mind, body or spirit: _____

Number of hours I rested or slept in past 24 hours:
____Rest   ____Sleep

Prayer/Meditation for the day:
☼ Yes   ☼ No

I am grateful for: _____

Today I did this one little thing
　　For the earth...
　　　　for a friend or a stranger...
　　　　　　for someone older or younger...
　　　　　　　　for someone sicker...
　　　　　　　　　　in more need... _____

September 15ᵀᴴ

❝*Worry does not empty tomorrow of its sorrow; it empties today of its strength.*❞
—CORRIE TEN BOOM

What are my biggest worries? What
will I gain from letting them go? _____

The best part of my day: _____

Something that made me laugh: _____

Whom did I let "off the hook" today? _____

Someone / Something that brings me joy: _____

Where kindness touched my world today: _____

How I nourished my mind, body or spirit: _____

Number of hours I rested or slept in past 24 hours:
___ Rest   ___ Sleep

Prayer/Meditation for the day:
☼ Yes   ☼ No

I am grateful for: _____

Today I did this one little thing
    For the earth...
        for a friend or a stranger...
            for someone older or younger...
                for someone sicker...
                    in more need... _____

> **"***It's not so much the hole inside me that I mind,***" she said. "***it's the weight that's in that hole.***" "***Then take the weight out and leave it behind and fill the hole with things that will make you fly,***" was her reply.**

—TERRI ST. CLOUD
BONESIGHARTS.COM

What quality do I most want
to share with the world? _____

The best part of my day: _____

Something that made me laugh: _____

Whom did I let "off the hook" today? _____

Someone / Something that brings me joy: _____

Where kindness touched my world today: _____

How I nourished my mind, body or spirit: _____

Number of hours I rested or slept in past 24 hours:
___ Rest   ___ Sleep

Prayer/Meditation for the day:
☼ Yes   ☼ No

I am grateful for: _____

Today I did this one little thing
    For the earth...
        for a friend or a stranger...
            for someone older or younger...
                for someone sicker...
                    in more need... _____

September 17TH

> *" The most beautiful things in the world cannot be seen*
> *or even touched, they must be felt with the heart. "*
> —HELEN KELLER

Something beautiful I have felt with my heart: _____

The best part of my day: _____

Something that made me laugh: _____

Whom did I let "off the hook" today? _____

Someone / Something that brings me joy: _____

Where kindness touched my world today: _____

How I nourished my mind, body or spirit: _____

Number of hours I rested or slept in past 24 hours:
___ Rest   ___ Sleep

Prayer/Meditation for the day:
☼ Yes   ☼ No

I am grateful for: _____

Today I did this one little thing
   For the earth...
      for a friend or a stranger...
         for someone older or younger...
           for someone sicker...
              in more need... _____

September 18TH

"Laughter is man's most distinctive emotional expression."
—MARGARET MEAD

What made me laugh today? _____

The best part of my day: _____

Something that made me laugh: _____

Whom did I let "off the hook" today? _____

Someone / Something that brings me joy: _____

Where kindness touched my world today: _____

How I nourished my mind, body or spirit: _____

Number of hours I rested or slept in past 24 hours:
___ Rest   ___ Sleep

Prayer/Meditation for the day:
☼ Yes   ☼ No

I am grateful for: _____

Today I did this one little thing
    For the earth...
        for a friend or a stranger...
            for someone older or younger...
                for someone sicker...
                    in more need... _____

September 19TH

> "*A smile is the beginning of peace.*"
> —MOTHER TERESA

I love: _____

The best part of my day: _____

Something that made me laugh: _____

Whom did I let "off the hook" today? _____

Someone / Something that brings me joy: _____

Where kindness touched my world today: _____

How I nourished my mind, body or spirit: _____

Number of hours I rested or slept in past 24 hours:
____ Rest   ____ Sleep

Prayer/Meditation for the day:
☼ Yes   ☼ No

I am grateful for: _____ , _____

Today I did this one little thing
   For the earth...
      for a friend or a stranger...
         for someone older or younger...
            for someone sicker...
               in more need... _____

> " *Not knowing when the dawn will come I open every door.* "
> —EMILY DICKINSON

What doors have I opened? _____

The best part of my day: _____

Something that made me laugh: _____

Whom did I let "off the hook" today? _____

Someone / Something that brings me joy: _____

Where kindness touched my world today: _____

How I nourished my mind, body or spirit: _____

Number of hours I rested or slept in past 24 hours:
___ Rest   ___ Sleep

Prayer/Meditation for the day:
☼ Yes   ☼ No

I am grateful for: _____

Today I did this one little thing
    For the earth...
        for a friend or a stranger...
            for someone older or younger...
                for someone sicker...
                    in more need... _____

Mid Month
Review

Best part of the past ten days? _____

Number of days I laughed: _____

Goal I want to set for the next 10 days: _____

Person/people who did or
said something to help me heal: _____

Anything else I have noticed
or want to remember/record: _____

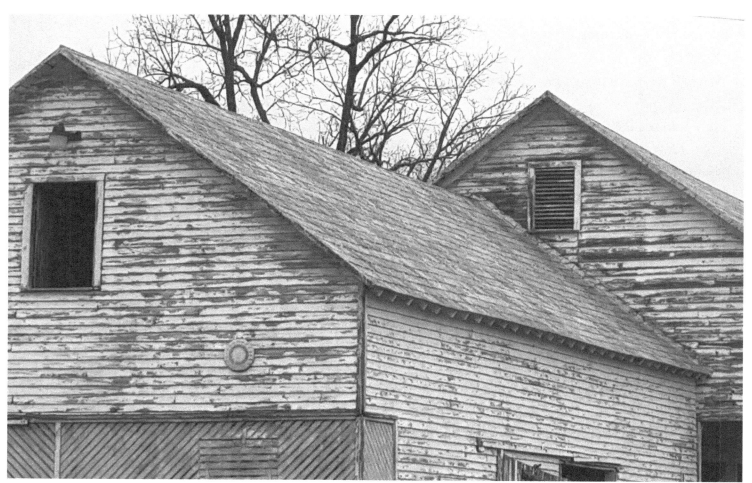

©ALYSSA KNAPP

September 21ST

"Our spiritual vision has to be cultivated. The ability to see the extraordinary in the ordinary needs to be recaptured and nurtured. It is valuable beyond wealth, because it gives us the ability to transform the dark into light."

—JEANNE SELANDER MILLER
A BREATH AWAY

What do I see as extraordinary today? _____

The best part of my day: _____

Something that made me laugh: _____

Whom did I let "off the hook" today? _____

Someone / Something that brings me joy: _____

Where kindness touched my world today: _____

How I nourished my mind, body or spirit: _____

Number of hours I rested or slept in past 24 hours:
___ Rest ___ Sleep

Prayer/Meditation for the day:
☼ Yes ☼ No

I am grateful for: _____

Today I did this one little thing
    For the earth...
        for a friend or a stranger...
            for someone older or younger...
                for someone sicker...
                    in more need... _____

September 22ND

> **"***Each day has a color, a smell.***"**
> —CHITRA BANERJEE DIVAKARUNI
> *THE MISTRESS OF SPICES*
> PENGUIN RANDOM HOUSE

Today, I smelled: _____

The best part of my day: _____

Something that made me laugh: _____

Whom did I let "off the hook" today? _____

Someone / Something that brings me joy: _____

Where kindness touched my world today: _____

How I nourished my mind, body or spirit: _____

Number of hours I rested or slept in past 24 hours:
___ Rest ___ Sleep

Prayer/Meditation for the day:
☼ Yes   ☼ No

I am grateful for: _____

Today I did this one little thing
    For the earth...
        for a friend or a stranger...
            for someone older or younger...
                for someone sicker...
                    in more need... _____

September 23RD

" *It is better to live your own destiny imperfectly than to live an imitation of somebody else's life with perfection.* **"**
—BHAGAVAD GITA

Today, I choose to: _____

The best part of my day: _____

Something that made me laugh: _____

Whom did I let "off the hook" today? _____

Someone / Something that brings me joy: _____

Where kindness touched my world today: _____

How I nourished my mind, body or spirit: _____

Number of hours I rested or slept in past 24 hours:
___ Rest   ___ Sleep

Prayer/Meditation for the day:
☀ Yes   ☀ No

I am grateful for: _____

Today I did this one little thing
For the earth...
for a friend or a stranger...
for someone older or younger...
for someone sicker...
in more need... _____

September 24TH

"*We never know which lives we influence, or when, or why.*"
—STEPHEN KING

Whose life have I influenced? _____

The best part of my day: _____

Something that made me laugh: _____

Whom did I let "off the hook" today? _____

Someone / Something that brings me joy: _____

Where kindness touched my world today: _____

How I nourished my mind, body or spirit: _____

Number of hours I rested or slept in past 24 hours:
___ Rest   ___ Sleep

Prayer/Meditation for the day:
☼ Yes   ☼ No

I am grateful for: _____

Today I did this one little thing
    For the earth...
        for a friend or a stranger...
           for someone older or younger...
             for someone sicker...
                in more need... _____

> **"***if i could teach you anything - it would be to hear your heart,
> and know your beauty and to believe in your possibilities.***"**
>
> —TERRI ST. CLOUD
> BONESIGHARTS.COM

Am I listening to my heart today? _____

The best part of my day: _____

Something that made me laugh: _____

Whom did I let "off the hook" today? _____

Someone / Something that brings me joy: _____

Where kindness touched my world today: _____

How I nourished my mind, body or spirit: _____

Number of hours I rested or slept in past 24 hours:
___Rest ___Sleep

Prayer/Meditation for the day:
☼ Yes ☼ No

I am grateful for: _____

Today I did this one little thing
    For the earth...
        for a friend or a stranger...
           for someone older or younger...
             for someone sicker...
               in more need... _____

September 26th

" Hug and kiss whoever helped get you - financially, mentally, morally, emotionally - to this day. Parents, mentors, friends, teachers. If you're too uptight to do that, at least do the old handshake thing, but I recommend a hug and a kiss. Don't let the sun go down without saying thank you to someone, and without admitting to yourself that absolutely no one gets this far alone."

—STEPHEN KING

Who did I hug and kiss today? _____

The best part of my day: _____

Something that made me laugh: _____

Whom did I let "off the hook" today? _____

Someone / Something that brings me joy: _____

Where kindness touched my world today: _____

How I nourished my mind, body or spirit: _____

Number of hours I rested or slept in past 24 hours:
___ Rest   ___ Sleep

Prayer/Meditation for the day:
☼ Yes   ☼ No

I am grateful for: _____

Today I did this one little thing
    For the earth...
        for a friend or a stranger...
            for someone older or younger...
                for someone sicker...
                    in more need... _____

September 27TH

" In wisdom gathered over time I have found
that every experience is a form of exploration."
—ANSEL ADAMS

I explored: _____

The best part of my day: _____

Something that made me laugh: _____

Whom did I let "off the hook" today? _____

Someone / Something that brings me joy: _____

Where kindness touched my world today: _____

How I nourished my mind, body or spirit: _____

Number of hours I rested or slept in past 24 hours:
___Rest ___Sleep

Prayer/Meditation for the day:
☀ Yes ☀ No

I am grateful for: _____

Today I did this one little thing
     For the earth...
          for a friend or a stranger...
               for someone older or younger...
                    for someone sicker...
                         in more need... _____

September 28TH

> "*Every trial endured and weathered in the right spirit*
> *makes a soul nobler and stronger than it was before.*"
> —JAMES BUCKHAM

I am trying to: _____

The best part of my day: _____

Something that made me laugh: _____

Whom did I let "off the hook" today? _____

Someone / Something that brings me joy: _____

Where kindness touched my world today: _____

How I nourished my mind, body or spirit: _____

Number of hours I rested or slept in past 24 hours:
___Rest   ___Sleep

Prayer/Meditation for the day:
☼ Yes   ☼ No

I am grateful for: _____

Today I did this one little thing
    For the earth...
        for a friend or a stranger...
            for someone older or younger...
                for someone sicker...
                    in more need... _____

September 29TH

❝*It is not balance you need but adaptability.***❞**
—ERWIN RAPHAEL MCMANUS
WIDE AWAKE: THE FUTURE IS WAITING WITHIN YOU

How I am adapting: _____

The best part of my day: _____

Something that made me laugh: _____

Whom did I let "off the hook" today? _____

Someone / Something that brings me joy: _____

Where kindness touched my world today: _____

How I nourished my mind, body or spirit: _____

Number of hours I rested or slept in past 24 hours:
___Rest   ___Sleep

Prayer/Meditation for the day:
☼ Yes   ☼ No

I am grateful for: _____

Today I did this one little thing
    For the earth...
        for a friend or a stranger...
           for someone older or younger...
             for someone sicker...
                in more need... _____

September 30TH

"We grow great by dreams. All big men are dreamers. They see things in the soft haze of a spring day or in the red fire of a long winter's evening. Some of us let these great dreams die, but others nourish and protect them; nurse them through bad days till they bring them to the sunshine and light which comes always to those who sincerely hope that their dreams will come true."

—WOODROW WILSON

I am planning to: _____

The best part of my day: _____

Something that made me laugh: _____

Whom did I let "off the hook" today? _____

Someone / Something that brings me joy: _____

Where kindness touched my world today: _____

How I nourished my mind, body or spirit: _____

Number of hours I rested or slept in past 24 hours:
___ Rest ___ Sleep

Prayer/Meditation for the day:
☼ Yes ☼ No

I am grateful for: _____

Today I did this one little thing
　　For the earth...
　　　　for a friend or a stranger...
　　　　　　for someone older or younger...
　　　　　　　　for someone sicker...
　　　　　　　　　　in more need... _____

End of Month Review

Best part of the past ten days? _____

Number of days I laughed: _____

Goal I want to set for the next 10 days: _____

Person/people who did or
said something to help me heal: _____

Anything else I have noticed
or want to remember/record: _____

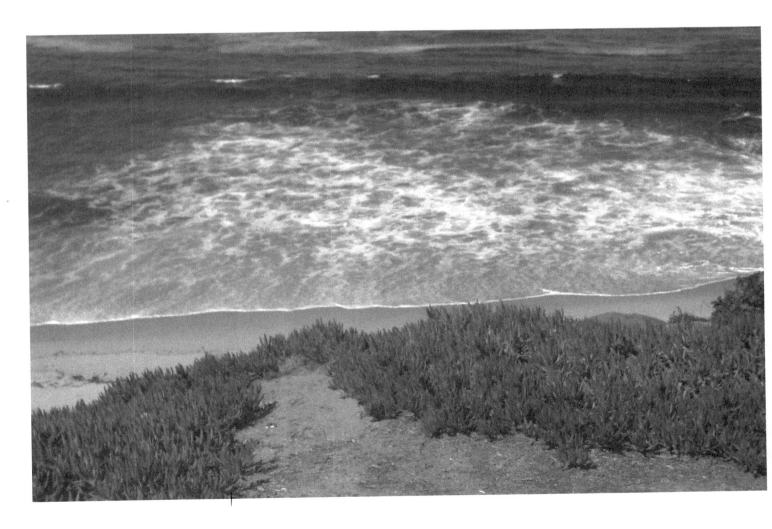

October 1ST

" The earth has music for those who listen. "
—GEORGE SANTAYANA

I love listening to: _____

The best part of my day: _____

Something that made me laugh: _____

Whom did I let "off the hook" today? _____

Someone / Something that brings me joy: _____

Where kindness touched my world today: _____

How I nourished my mind, body or spirit: _____

Number of hours I rested or slept in past 24 hours:
___ Rest ___ Sleep

Prayer/Meditation for the day:
☼ Yes   ☼ No

I am grateful for: _____

Today I did this one little thing
    For the earth...
        for a friend or a stranger...
            for someone older or younger...
                for someone sicker...
                    in more need... _____

> " *Courage is fear that has said its prayers.* "
> —ANONYMOUS

I am comforted by: _____

The best part of my day: _____

Something that made me laugh: _____

Whom did I let "off the hook" today? _____

Someone / Something that brings me joy: _____

Where kindness touched my world today: _____

How I nourished my mind, body or spirit: _____

Number of hours I rested or slept in past 24 hours:
___ Rest   ___ Sleep

Prayer/Meditation for the day:
☼ Yes   ☼ No

I am grateful for: _____

Today I did this one little thing
   For the earth...
      for a friend or a stranger...
         for someone older or younger...
           for someone sicker...
              in more need... _____

October 3RD

"Asking for help is part of the healing process."
—SHARON RAINEY

Did I ask for help today? _____

The best part of my day: _____

Something that made me laugh: _____

Whom did I let "off the hook" today? _____

Someone / Something that brings me joy: _____

Where kindness touched my world today: _____

How I nourished my mind, body or spirit: _____

Number of hours I rested or slept in past 24 hours:
___ Rest   ___ Sleep

Prayer/Meditation for the day:
☼ Yes   ☼ No

I am grateful for: _____

Today I did this one little thing
    For the earth...
        for a friend or a stranger...
            for someone older or younger...
                for someone sicker...
                    in more need... _____

> " *The first step towards getting somewhere is to
> decide that you are not going to stay where you are.* "
> —ANONYMOUS

Something I want to let go of: _____

The best part of my day: _____

Something that made me laugh: _____

Whom did I let "off the hook" today? _____

Someone / Something that brings me joy: _____

Where kindness touched my world today: _____

How I nourished my mind, body or spirit: _____

Number of hours I rested or slept in past 24 hours:
___ Rest ___ Sleep

Prayer/Meditation for the day:
☼ Yes   ☼ No

I am grateful for: _____

Today I did this one little thing
　　For the earth...
　　　　for a friend or a stranger...
　　　　　　for someone older or younger...
　　　　　　　　for someone sicker...
　　　　　　　　　　in more need... _____

October 5TH

> " *Courage doesn't always roar. Sometimes courage is the quiet voice at the end of the day saying, I will try again tomorrow.* "
> —MARY ANN RADMACHER
> *LIFE BEGINS WHEN YOU DO*

I said no to: _____

The best part of my day: _____

Something that made me laugh: _____

Whom did I let "off the hook" today? _____

Someone / Something that brings me joy: _____

Where kindness touched my world today: _____

How I nourished my mind, body or spirit: _____

Number of hours I rested or slept in past 24 hours:
___ Rest   ___ Sleep

Prayer/Meditation for the day:
☼ Yes   ☼ No

I am grateful for: _____

Today I did this one little thing
    For the earth...
        for a friend or a stranger...
            for someone older or younger...
                for someone sicker...
                    in more need... _____

October 6TH

" *You have been offered "the gift of crisis." As Kathleen Norris reminds us, the Greek root of the word crisis is "to sift", as in, to shake out the excesses and leave only what's important. That's what crises do. They shake things up until we are forced to hold on to only what matters most. The rest falls away.* "

—GLENNON DOYLE MELTON

CARRY ON, WARRIOR: THE POWER OF EMBRACING YOUR MESSY, BEAUTIFUL LIFE

What am I willing to shake out of my life today? _____

The best part of my day: _____

Something that made me laugh: _____

Whom did I let "off the hook" today? _____

Someone / Something that brings me joy: _____

Where kindness touched my world today: _____

How I nourished my mind, body or spirit: _____

Number of hours I rested or slept in past 24 hours:
___ Rest   ___ Sleep

Prayer/Meditation for the day:
☼ Yes   ☼ No

I am grateful for: _____

Today I did this one little thing
    For the earth...
        for a friend or a stranger...
            for someone older or younger...
                for someone sicker...
                    in more need... _____

October 7TH

> "*I am not afraid of storms, for I am learning how to sail my ship.*"
> —LOUISA MAY ALCOTT

How I am preparing for the next storm
and what is my next storm? Do I know? _____

The best part of my day: _____

Something that made me laugh: _____

Whom did I let "off the hook" today? _____

Someone / Something that brings me joy: _____

Where kindness touched my world today: _____

How I nourished my mind, body or spirit: _____

Number of hours I rested or slept in past 24 hours:
___ Rest   ___ Sleep

Prayer/Meditation for the day:
☼ Yes   ☼ No

I am grateful for: _____

Today I did this one little thing
　　For the earth...
　　　　for a friend or a stranger...
　　　　　　for someone older or younger...
　　　　　　　　for someone sicker...
　　　　　　　　　　in more need... _____

> "*Anger can be utilized to energize resolve and determination.*"
> —DAVID HAWKINS, MD
> *HEALING AND RECOVERY*

Today, I am determined to: _____

The best part of my day: _____

Something that made me laugh: _____

Whom did I let "off the hook" today? _____

Someone / Something that brings me joy: _____

Where kindness touched my world today: _____

How I nourished my mind, body or spirit: _____

Number of hours I rested or slept in past 24 hours:
___ Rest ___ Sleep

Prayer/Meditation for the day:
☼ Yes ☼ No

I am grateful for: _____

Today I did this one little thing
    For the earth...
        for a friend or a stranger...
           for someone older or younger...
              for someone sicker...
                in more need... _____

October 9ᵀᴴ

"Waiting is not my strength but, often it's necessary, to grow the strength I need."
—LYNDA DAVIS

How waiting has helped me grow stronger: _____

The best part of my day: _____

Something that made me laugh: _____

Whom did I let "off the hook" today? _____

Someone / Something that brings me joy: _____

Where kindness touched my world today: _____

How I nourished my mind, body or spirit: _____

Number of hours I rested or slept in past 24 hours:
___ Rest   ___ Sleep

Prayer/Meditation for the day:
☼ Yes   ☼ No

I am grateful for: _____

Today I did this one little thing
    For the earth...
        for a friend or a stranger...
           for someone older or younger...
              for someone sicker...
                in more need... _____

> " *Perhaps power is letting go of the grip of the past*
> *and standing empty handed facing the future.* "
> —TERRI ST. CLOUD
> BONESIGHARTS.COM

What is holding me back from moving on? How
can I let go and let myself be "empty handed?" _____

The best part of my day: _____

Something that made me laugh: _____

Whom did I let "off the hook" today? _____

Someone / Something that brings me joy: _____

Where kindness touched my world today: _____

How I nourished my mind, body or spirit: _____

Number of hours I rested or slept in past 24 hours:
___Rest   ___Sleep

Prayer/Meditation for the day:
☼ Yes   ☼ No

I am grateful for: _____

Today I did this one little thing
    For the earth...
        for a friend or a stranger...
            for someone older or younger...
                for someone sicker...
                    in more need... _____

Early Month Review

Best part of the past ten days? _____

Number of days I laughed: _____

Goal I want to set for the next 10 days: _____

Person/people who did or
said something to help me heal: _____

Anything else I have noticed
or want to remember/record: _____

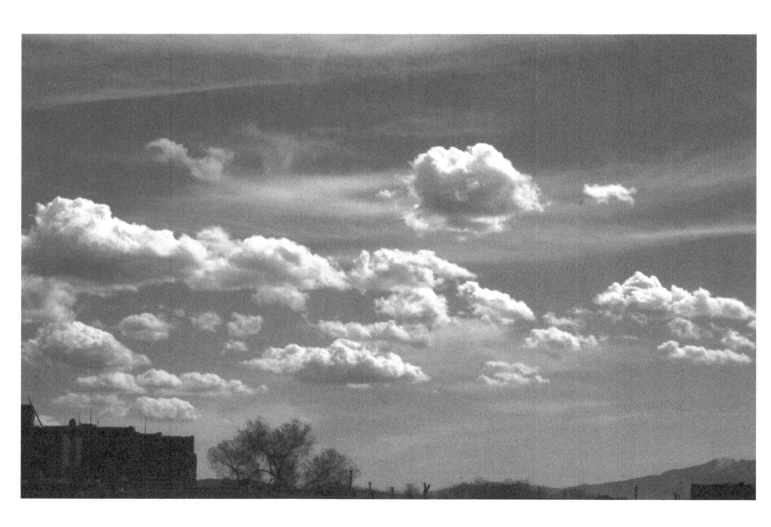

> " *People talk about love as though it were something you could give, like an armful of flowers. And a lot of people give love like that, just dump it down on top of you, a useless, strong-scented burden. I don't think it is anything you can give. Love is a force in you that enables you to give other things. It is the motivating power. It enables you to give strength and power and freedom and peace to another person. It is not a result; it is a cause. It is not a product; it produces. It is a power, like money, or steam or electricity. It is valueless unless you can give something else by means of it.* "
> —ANNE MORROW LINDBERGH

How has love affected my healing? _____

The best part of my day: _____

Something that made me laugh: _____

Whom did I let "off the hook" today? _____

Someone / Something that brings me joy: _____

Where kindness touched my world today: _____

How I nourished my mind, body or spirit: _____

Number of hours I rested or slept in past 24 hours:
___Rest ___Sleep

Prayer/Meditation for the day:
☼ Yes ☼ No

I am grateful for: _____

Today I did this one little thing
 For the earth...
  for a friend or a stranger...
   for someone older or younger...
    for someone sicker...
     in more need... _____

October 12ᵀᴴ

" *For us there is only the trying. The rest is not our business.* "
—T.S. ELIOT

I listened to my body today: ☼ Yes ☼ No

The best part of my day: _____

Something that made me laugh: _____

Whom did I let "off the hook" today? _____

Someone / Something that brings me joy: _____

Where kindness touched my world today: _____

How I nourished my mind, body or spirit: _____

Number of hours I rested or slept in past 24 hours:
___ Rest ___ Sleep

Prayer/Meditation for the day:
☼ Yes ☼ No

I am grateful for: _____

Today I did this one little thing
    For the earth...
        for a friend or a stranger...
            for someone older or younger...
                for someone sicker...
                    in more need... _____

> **"** *I thrive in a place of love and goodness. So my focus will continue to be on surrounding myself with goodness and creating boundaries from the unfriendliness in this world.* **"**
> —ALYSSA KNAPP

What people and things do I surround myself with? Does the joy I get from them outweigh the negativity in the world? _____

The best part of my day: _____

Something that made me laugh: _____

Whom did I let "off the hook" today? _____

Someone / Something that brings me joy: _____

Where kindness touched my world today: _____

How I nourished my mind, body or spirit: _____

Number of hours I rested or slept in past 24 hours:
____Rest   ____Sleep

Prayer/Meditation for the day:
☼ Yes   ☼ No

I am grateful for: _____

Today I did this one little thing
    For the earth...
        for a friend or a stranger...
            for someone older or younger...
                for someone sicker...
                    in more need... _____

October 14TH

"Happiness is a choice, and though my body may never heal, I try every day to live as full a life as I am able. I choose to be happy."
—NULLIE STOCKTON

I felt happy today when: _____

The best part of my day: _____

Something that made me laugh: _____

Whom did I let "off the hook" today? _____

Someone / Something that brings me joy: _____

Where kindness touched my world today: _____

How I nourished my mind, body or spirit: _____

Number of hours I rested or slept in past 24 hours:
___ Rest   ___ Sleep

Prayer/Meditation for the day:
☼ Yes   ☼ No

I am grateful for: _____

Today I did this one little thing
    For the earth...
        for a friend or a stranger...
            for someone older or younger...
                for someone sicker...
                    in more need... _____

> " *One learns a good deal in the school of suffering. I wonder what would have happened to me if I had had an easy life, and had not had the privilege of tasting the joys of jail and all it means.* "
> —EKNATH EASWARAN

I am now free of: _____

The best part of my day: _____

Something that made me laugh: _____

Whom did I let "off the hook" today? _____

Someone / Something that brings me joy: _____

Where kindness touched my world today: _____

How I nourished my mind, body or spirit: _____

Number of hours I rested or slept in past 24 hours:
___ Rest ___ Sleep

Prayer/Meditation for the day:
☼ Yes ☼ No

I am grateful for: _____

Today I did this one little thing
    For the earth...
        for a friend or a stranger...
            for someone older or younger...
                for someone sicker...
                    in more need... _____

October 16TH

> " *There are, in fact, certain roads that one may follow. Simplification of life is one of them.* "
> —ANNE MORROW LINDBERGH

How have I simplified my life? _____

The best part of my day: _____

Something that made me laugh: _____

Whom did I let "off the hook" today? _____

Someone / Something that brings me joy: _____

Where kindness touched my world today: _____

How I nourished my mind, body or spirit: _____

Number of hours I rested or slept in past 24 hours:
___ Rest ___ Sleep

Prayer/Meditation for the day:
☼ Yes ☼ No

I am grateful for: _____

Today I did this one little thing
    For the earth...
        for a friend or a stranger...
           for someone older or younger...
             for someone sicker...
                in more need... _____

" One and one and one and one doesn't equal four. Each one remains unique, there is no way of joining them together. They cannot be exchanged, one for the other. They cannot replace each other."
—MARGARET ATWOOD

Who is irreplaceable in my life and why: _____

The best part of my day: _____

Something that made me laugh: _____

Whom did I let "off the hook" today? _____

Someone / Something that brings me joy: _____

Where kindness touched my world today: _____

How I nourished my mind, body or spirit: _____

Number of hours I rested or slept in past 24 hours:
___ Rest ___ Sleep

Prayer/Meditation for the day:
☼ Yes ☼ No

I am grateful for: _____

Today I did this one little thing
For the earth...
for a friend or a stranger...
for someone older or younger...
for someone sicker...
in more need... _____

October 18TH

" Dreams are illustrations from the book your soul is writing about you."
—MARSHA NORMAN

My soul dreams of: _____

The best part of my day: _____

Something that made me laugh: _____

Whom did I let "off the hook" today? _____

Someone / Something that brings me joy: _____

Where kindness touched my world today: _____

How I nourished my mind, body or spirit: _____

Number of hours I rested or slept in past 24 hours:
____ Rest   ____ Sleep

Prayer/Meditation for the day:
☼ Yes   ☼ No

I am grateful for: _____

Today I did this one little thing
    For the earth...
        for a friend or a stranger...
           for someone older or younger...
              for someone sicker...
                in more need... _____

> **❝** *To get joy, we must give it, and to keep joy, we must scatter it.* **❞**
> —JOHN TEMPLETON

I am excited about: _____

The best part of my day: _____

Something that made me laugh: _____

Whom did I let "off the hook" today? _____

Someone / Something that brings me joy: _____

Where kindness touched my world today: _____

How I nourished my mind, body or spirit: _____

Number of hours I rested or slept in past 24 hours:
___ Rest   ___ Sleep

Prayer/Meditation for the day:
☼ Yes   ☼ No

I am grateful for: _____

Today I did this one little thing
    For the earth...
        for a friend or a stranger...
           for someone older or younger...
             for someone sicker...
               in more need... _____

October 20TH

> **"** *Put your ear down close to your soul and listen hard.* **"**
> —ANNE SEXTON

What I heard when I listened hard: _____

The best part of my day: _____

Something that made me laugh: _____

Whom did I let "off the hook" today? _____

Someone / Something that brings me joy: _____

Where kindness touched my world today: _____

How I nourished my mind, body or spirit: _____

Number of hours I rested or slept in past 24 hours:
___ Rest   ___ Sleep

Prayer/Meditation for the day:
☼ Yes   ☼ No

I am grateful for: _____

Today I did this one little thing
    For the earth...
        for a friend or a stranger...
            for someone older or younger...
                for someone sicker...
                    in more need... _____

Mid Month Review

Best part of the past ten days? _____

Number of days I laughed: _____

Goal I want to set for the next 10 days: _____

Person/people who did or
said something to help me heal: _____

Anything else I have noticed
or want to remember/record: _____

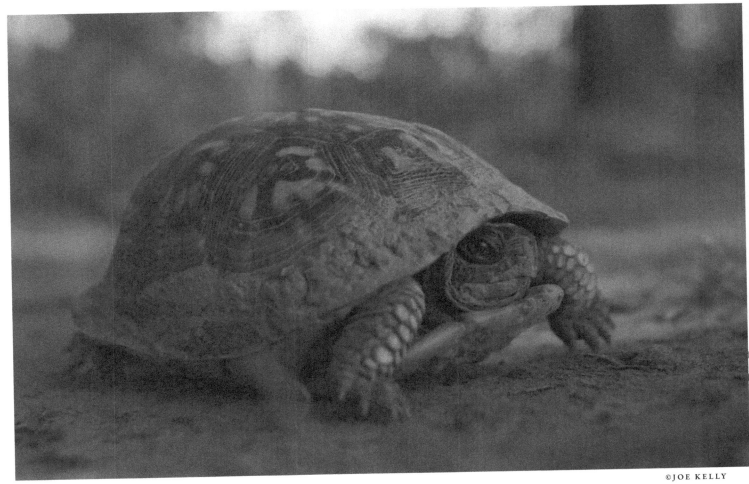

©JOE KELLY

October 21ST

> " *Telling the truth is simplicity itself, and with it comes an avalanche of relief. Now I understand that bringing your secrets out into the bright sunlight instantly removes their dark power.* "
> —KRISTEN JOHNSTON
> *GUTS: THE ENDLESS FOLLIES AND TINY TRIUMPHS OF A GIANT DISASTER*

I am excited about: _____

The best part of my day: _____

Something that made me laugh: _____

Whom did I let "off the hook" today? _____

Someone / Something that brings me joy: _____

Where kindness touched my world today: _____

How I nourished my mind, body or spirit: _____

Number of hours I rested or slept in past 24 hours:
___ Rest   ___ Sleep

Prayer/Meditation for the day:
☼ Yes   ☼ No

I am grateful for: _____

Today I did this one little thing
    For the earth...
        for a friend or a stranger...
            for someone older or younger...
                for someone sicker...
                    in more need... _____

October 22ND

"Knowledge of what is possible is the beginning of happiness."
—GEORGE SANTAYANA

Do I want to be right or do I want to be happy? _____

The best part of my day: _____

Something that made me laugh: _____

Whom did I let "off the hook" today? _____

Someone / Something that brings me joy: _____

Where kindness touched my world today: _____

How I nourished my mind, body or spirit: _____

Number of hours I rested or slept in past 24 hours:
___ Rest ___ Sleep

Prayer/Meditation for the day:
☼ Yes   ☼ No

I am grateful for: _____

Today I did this one little thing
    For the earth...
        for a friend or a stranger...
            for someone older or younger...
                for someone sicker...
                    in more need... _____

October 23RD

> **"** *The body does not heal in chaos. The body only heals in peace.* **"**
> —DOLORES CANNON
> *THE THREE WAVES OF VOLUNTEERS*

Am I creating a place for my body to heal? _____

The best part of my day: _____

Something that made me laugh: _____

Whom did I let "off the hook" today? _____

Someone / Something that brings me joy: _____

Where kindness touched my world today: _____

How I nourished my mind, body or spirit: _____

Number of hours I rested or slept in past 24 hours:
___ Rest   ___ Sleep

Prayer/Meditation for the day:
☼ Yes   ☼ No

I am grateful for: _____

Today I did this one little thing
    For the earth...
        for a friend or a stranger...
            for someone older or younger...
                for someone sicker...
                    in more need... _____

October 24TH

> " *The ultimate measure of a man is not where he stands in moments of comfort and convenience, but where he stands at times of challenge and controversy.* "
> —MARTIN LUTHER KING, JR.

One of my recent challenging episodes: _____

The best part of my day: _____

Something that made me laugh: _____

Whom did I let "off the hook" today? _____

Someone / Something that brings me joy: _____

Where kindness touched my world today: _____

How I nourished my mind, body or spirit: _____

Number of hours I rested or slept in past 24 hours:
___Rest   ___Sleep

Prayer/Meditation for the day:
☼ Yes   ☼ No

I am grateful for: _____

Today I did this one little thing
    For the earth...
        for a friend or a stranger...
            for someone older or younger...
                for someone sicker...
                    in more need... _____

October 25ᴛʜ

"You cannot swim for new horizons until you have courage to lose sight of the shore."
—WILLIAM FAULKNER

Something I haven't let go of: _____

The best part of my day: _____

Something that made me laugh: _____

Whom did I let "off the hook" today? _____

Someone / Something that brings me joy: _____

Where kindness touched my world today: _____

How I nourished my mind, body or spirit: _____

Number of hours I rested or slept in past 24 hours:
___ Rest   ___ Sleep

Prayer/Meditation for the day:
☼ Yes   ☼ No

I am grateful for: _____

Today I did this one little thing
    For the earth...
        for a friend or a stranger...
            for someone older or younger...
                for someone sicker...
                    in more need... _____

"As we balance and become more and more identified with our spiritual nature, and the ego returns to its designated place, we again are led by the Spirit, but now in a conscious way."

—GERRY BOYLAN

WHAT ARE YOU HOLDING ONTO THAT'S HOLDING YOU BACK?

Who/What gave me energy today: _____

The best part of my day: _____

Something that made me laugh: _____

Whom did I let "off the hook" today? _____

Someone / Something that brings me joy: _____

Where kindness touched my world today: _____

How I nourished my mind, body or spirit: _____

Number of hours I rested or slept in past 24 hours:
___Rest   ___Sleep

Prayer/Meditation for the day:
☼ Yes   ☼ No

I am grateful for: _____

Today I did this one little thing
    For the earth...
        for a friend or a stranger...
            for someone older or younger...
                for someone sicker...
                    in more need... _____

October 27TH

"*Even if you are a minority of one, the truth is the truth.***"**
—MAHATMA GANDHI

A truth I now can say out loud: _____

The best part of my day: _____

Something that made me laugh: _____

Whom did I let "off the hook" today? _____

Someone / Something that brings me joy: _____

Where kindness touched my world today: _____

How I nourished my mind, body or spirit: _____

Number of hours I rested or slept in past 24 hours:
___Rest ___Sleep

Prayer/Meditation for the day:
☼ Yes ☼ No

I am grateful for: _____

Today I did this one little thing
    For the earth...
        for a friend or a stranger...
            for someone older or younger...
                for someone sicker...
                    in more need... _____

October 28TH

" True happiness is proportional only to my yielding to the brokenness, and not to my refusing to accept it or to my struggling to overcome it. "
—DAVID PATTEN

Today, I accept: _____

The best part of my day: _____

Something that made me laugh: _____

Whom did I let "off the hook" today? _____

Someone / Something that brings me joy: _____

Where kindness touched my world today: _____

How I nourished my mind, body or spirit: _____

Number of hours I rested or slept in past 24 hours:
___Rest ___Sleep

Prayer/Meditation for the day:
☼ Yes ☼ No

I am grateful for: _____

Today I did this one little thing
    For the earth...
        for a friend or a stranger...
           for someone older or younger...
              for someone sicker...
                in more need... _____

October 29TH

"Solitary trees, if they grow at all, grow strong."
—WINSTON CHURCHILL

Something that made me feel good today: _____

The best part of my day: _____

Something that made me laugh: _____

Whom did I let "off the hook" today? _____

Someone / Something that brings me joy: _____

Where kindness touched my world today: _____

How I nourished my mind, body or spirit: _____

Number of hours I rested or slept in past 24 hours:
___ Rest   ___ Sleep

Prayer/Meditation for the day:
☼ Yes   ☼ No

I am grateful for: _____

Today I did this one little thing
   For the earth...
      for a friend or a stranger...
         for someone older or younger...
           for someone sicker...
              in more need... _____

> **"** *Masaru Emoto's photographs of water crystals were featured in a documentary. They showed how water spoken to with positive words formed complete, beautiful crystals. Water spoken angry words to formed distorted crystals. Our bodies are 70% water. What are our words doing to us?* **"**
> —SHARON RAINEY

What loving, positive words have I spoken today? _____

The best part of my day: _____

Something that made me laugh: _____

Whom did I let "off the hook" today? _____

Someone / Something that brings me joy: _____

Where kindness touched my world today: _____

How I nourished my mind, body or spirit: _____

Number of hours I rested or slept in past 24 hours:
____ Rest   ____ Sleep

Prayer/Meditation for the day:
☼ Yes   ☼ No

I am grateful for: _____

Today I did this one little thing
    For the earth...
        for a friend or a stranger...
           for someone older or younger...
               for someone sicker...
                  in more need... _____

October 31ST

> *"Our experiences affect our biology, particularly when these experiences are chronic, happen early in life, and remain unrecognized."*
> —ROBIN KARR-MORSE
> *SCARED SICK: THE ROLE OF CHILDHOOD TRAUMA IN ADULT DISEASE*

What remained unrecognized in my life? _____

The best part of my day: _____

Something that made me laugh: _____

Whom did I let "off the hook" today? _____

Someone / Something that brings me joy: _____

Where kindness touched my world today: _____

How I nourished my mind, body or spirit: _____

Number of hours I rested or slept in past 24 hours:
___ Rest   ___ Sleep

Prayer/Meditation for the day:
☼ Yes   ☼ No

I am grateful for: _____

Today I did this one little thing
    For the earth...
        for a friend or a stranger...
           for someone older or younger...
             for someone sicker...
                in more need... _____

End of Month Review

Best part of the past ten days? _____

Number of days I laughed: _____

Goal I want to set for the next 10 days: _____

Person/people who did or
said something to help me heal: _____

Anything else I have noticed
or want to remember/record: _____

November 1ST

> *"Lives fall apart when they need to be rebuilt."*
> —IYANLA VANZANT

What I helped rebuild: _____

The best part of my day: _____

Something that made me laugh: _____

Whom did I let "off the hook" today? _____

Someone / Something that brings me joy: _____

Where kindness touched my world today: _____

How I nourished my mind, body or spirit: _____

Number of hours I rested or slept in past 24 hours:
____ Rest   ____ Sleep

Prayer/Meditation for the day:
☼ Yes   ☼ No

I am grateful for: _____

Today I did this one little thing
    For the earth...
        for a friend or a stranger...
            for someone older or younger...
                for someone sicker...
                    in more need... _____

> " *During deep meditation, I would occasionally hear a soothing voice outside of my own reassuring me that all would be okay in the end. There is no way to know whose voice was calling out in the midst of meditation, nor does it really matter. My personal belief is that these messages were emanating from my soul, directly linked to the divine. The messages served their purpose and were healing, empowering.* "
>
> —DR. NEIL SPECTOR

What message is my soul
communicating to me today? _____

The best part of my day: _____

Something that made me laugh: _____

Whom did I let "off the hook" today? _____

Someone / Something that brings me joy: _____

Where kindness touched my world today: _____

How I nourished my mind, body or spirit: _____

Number of hours I rested or slept in past 24 hours:
___ Rest ___ Sleep

Prayer/Meditation for the day:
☼ Yes ☼ No

I am grateful for: _____

Today I did this one little thing
    For the earth...
        for a friend or a stranger...
           for someone older or younger...
               for someone sicker...
                  in more need... _____

November 3RD

"Everything is possible. The impossible just takes longer."
—DAN BROWN
FROM DIGITAL FORTRESS © 1998 BY DAN BROWN.
REPRINTED BY PERMISSION OF ST. MARTIN'S PRESS. ALL RIGHTS RESERVED.

Something I previously thought was
impossible but now know is possible: _____

The best part of my day: _____

Something that made me laugh: _____

Whom did I let "off the hook" today? _____

Someone / Something that brings me joy: _____

Where kindness touched my world today: _____

How I nourished my mind, body or spirit: _____

Number of hours I rested or slept in past 24 hours:
___ Rest   ___ Sleep

Prayer/Meditation for the day:
☼ Yes   ☼ No

I am grateful for: _____

Today I did this one little thing
    For the earth...
        for a friend or a stranger...
            for someone older or younger...
                for someone sicker...
                    in more need... _____

" *My mistakes do not define my life.* "
—SHARON RAINEY
MAKING A PEARL FROM THE GRIT OF LIFE

Something I am doing right: _____

The best part of my day: _____

Something that made me laugh: _____

Whom did I let "off the hook" today? _____

Someone / Something that brings me joy: _____

Where kindness touched my world today: _____

How I nourished my mind, body or spirit: _____

Number of hours I rested or slept in past 24 hours:
___ Rest ___ Sleep

Prayer/Meditation for the day:
☼ Yes ☼ No

I am grateful for: _____

Today I did this one little thing
    For the earth...
        for a friend or a stranger...
           for someone older or younger...
             for someone sicker...
               in more need... _____

November 5TH

> *"Healing is the result of not just clinical processes but also of overall biological potentialities that often do not materialize without the unseen power of spiritual alignment."*
> —DAVID HAWKINS, MD
> *HEALING AND RECOVERY*

How I nourished my spirit today: _____

The best part of my day: _____

Something that made me laugh: _____

Whom did I let "off the hook" today? _____

Someone / Something that brings me joy: _____

Where kindness touched my world today: _____

How I nourished my mind, body or spirit: _____

Number of hours I rested or slept in past 24 hours:
___ Rest   ___ Sleep

Prayer/Meditation for the day:
☼ Yes   ☼ No

I am grateful for: _____

Today I did this one little thing
    For the earth...
        for a friend or a stranger...
            for someone older or younger...
                for someone sicker...
                    in more need... _____

" *I can only do what I can only do.* **"**
—SCOTT EASTWOOD

How I accepted my limitations recently: _____

The best part of my day: _____

Something that made me laugh: _____

Whom did I let "off the hook" today? _____

Someone / Something that brings me joy: _____

Where kindness touched my world today: _____

How I nourished my mind, body or spirit: _____

Number of hours I rested or slept in past 24 hours:
___ Rest ___ Sleep

Prayer/Meditation for the day:
☼ Yes ☼ No

I am grateful for: _____

Today I did this one little thing
    For the earth...
        for a friend or a stranger...
           for someone older or younger...
              for someone sicker...
                in more need... _____

November 7TH

> *"You do not need to know precisely what is happening, or exactly where it is all going. What you need is to recognize the possibilities and challenges offered by the present moment, and to embrace them with courage, faith and hope."*
> —THOMAS MERTON

What am I embracing with
courage, faith and hope? _____

The best part of my day: _____

Something that made me laugh: _____

Whom did I let "off the hook" today? _____

Someone / Something that brings me joy: _____

Where kindness touched my world today: _____

How I nourished my mind, body or spirit: _____

Number of hours I rested or slept in past 24 hours:
___ Rest   ___ Sleep

Prayer/Meditation for the day:
☼ Yes   ☼ No

I am grateful for: _____

Today I did this one little thing
    For the earth...
        for a friend or a stranger...
           for someone older or younger...
              for someone sicker...
                in more need... _____

"When you stretch yourself thin and you neglect your self-care... you lose sleep, you walk around on edge, you get frustrated with others when they take your time, and emotions, like loneliness and self-doubt, become magnified."

—ROBIN SHIRLEY
CLUBTBYH.COM/ABOUT-ROBIN-SHIRLEY

Today, I will show self care by: _____

The best part of my day: _____

Something that made me laugh: _____

Whom did I let "off the hook" today? _____

Someone / Something that brings me joy: _____

Where kindness touched my world today: _____

How I nourished my mind, body or spirit: _____

Number of hours I rested or slept in past 24 hours:
___ Rest   ___ Sleep

Prayer/Meditation for the day:
☼ Yes   ☼ No

I am grateful for: _____

Today I did this one little thing
 For the earth...
  for a friend or a stranger...
   for someone older or younger...
    for someone sicker...
     in more need... _____

November 9TH

" There's a crack (or cracks) in everyone... that's how the light of God gets in. "
—ELIZABETH GILBERT

A crack where I let the light of God in: _____

The best part of my day: _____

Something that made me laugh: _____

Whom did I let "off the hook" today? _____

Someone / Something that brings me joy: _____

Where kindness touched my world today: _____

How I nourished my mind, body or spirit: _____

Number of hours I rested or slept in past 24 hours:
____ Rest   ____ Sleep

Prayer/Meditation for the day:
☼ Yes   ☼ No

I am grateful for: _____

Today I did this one little thing
    For the earth...
        for a friend or a stranger...
            for someone older or younger...
                for someone sicker...
                    in more need... _____

> " *Plunging her hands deep into the mire, she touched her river of steel.*
> *shoving the muck out of the way, she let its silver waters cleanse her.* "
> —TERRI ST. CLOUD
> BONESIGHARTS.COM

I feel better when: _____

The best part of my day: _____

Something that made me laugh: _____

Whom did I let "off the hook" today? _____

Someone / Something that brings me joy: _____

Where kindness touched my world today: _____

How I nourished my mind, body or spirit: _____

Number of hours I rested or slept in past 24 hours:
___Rest   ___Sleep

Prayer/Meditation for the day:
☼ Yes   ☼ No

I am grateful for: _____

Today I did this one little thing
    For the earth...
        for a friend or a stranger...
            for someone older or younger...
                for someone sicker...
                    in more need... _____

Early Month Review

Best part of the past ten days? _____

Number of days I laughed: _____

Goal I want to set for the next 10 days: _____

Person/people who did or
said something to help me heal: _____

Anything else I have noticed
or want to remember/record: _____

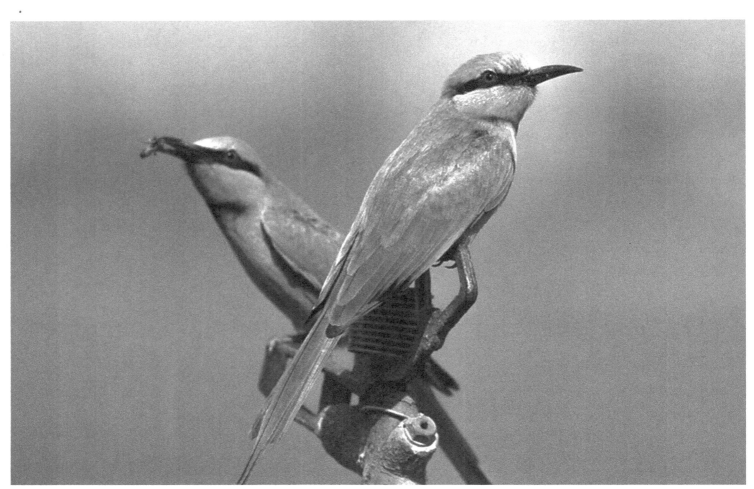

©JOE KELLY

November 11TH

" There's more beauty in truth, even if it is dreadful beauty. "
—JOHN STEINBECK

What truth do I know today
that may not be beautiful? _____

The best part of my day: _____

Something that made me laugh: _____

Whom did I let "off the hook" today? _____

Someone / Something that brings me joy: _____

Where kindness touched my world today: _____

How I nourished my mind, body or spirit: _____

Number of hours I rested or slept in past 24 hours:
____Rest   ____Sleep

Prayer/Meditation for the day:
☼ Yes   ☼ No

I am grateful for: _____

Today I did this one little thing
    For the earth...
        for a friend or a stranger...
            for someone older or younger...
                for someone sicker...
                    in more need... _____

November 12TH

> **"** *If we put half the effort we put into taking care of others, into taking care of ourselves, we might be healed by now. We avoid dealing with our own issues by putting all of our energy into others.* **"**
> —DEB JANSEN

Am I helping myself or am I helping
others and avoiding my own issues? _____

The best part of my day: _____

Something that made me laugh: _____

Whom did I let "off the hook" today? _____

Someone / Something that brings me joy: _____

Where kindness touched my world today: _____

How I nourished my mind, body or spirit: _____

Number of hours I rested or slept in past 24 hours:
___ Rest ___ Sleep

Prayer/Meditation for the day:
☼ Yes ☼ No

I am grateful for: _____

Today I did this one little thing
    For the earth...
        for a friend or a stranger...
            for someone older or younger...
                for someone sicker...
                    in more need... _____

November 13TH

"Just do you today."
—INDIA ARIE

How I am "doing me" today: _____

The best part of my day: _____

Something that made me laugh: _____

Whom did I let "off the hook" today? _____

Someone / Something that brings me joy: _____

Where kindness touched my world today: _____

How I nourished my mind, body or spirit: _____

Number of hours I rested or slept in past 24 hours:
___Rest   ___Sleep

Prayer/Meditation for the day:
☼ Yes   ☼ No

I am grateful for: _____

Today I did this one little thing
  For the earth...
    for a friend or a stranger...
      for someone older or younger...
        for someone sicker...
          in more need... _____

November 14TH

" The truth is life is full of joy and full of great
sorrow, but you can't have one without the other. "
—ANDRE DUBUS III

Can I see the balance in life today? _____

The best part of my day: _____

Something that made me laugh: _____

Whom did I let "off the hook" today? _____

Someone / Something that brings me joy: _____

Where kindness touched my world today: _____

How I nourished my mind, body or spirit: _____

Number of hours I rested or slept in past 24 hours:
___ Rest   ___ Sleep

Prayer/Meditation for the day:
☼ Yes   ☼ No

I am grateful for: _____

Today I did this one little thing
    For the earth...
        for a friend or a stranger...
            for someone older or younger...
                for someone sicker...
                    in more need... _____

November 15TH

"Sometimes compassion comes in the form of just sitting in someone's darkest room with them, knowing that the only promise in life is that our own rooms will one day go dark, as well."
—AMY MONTICELLO

Someone I could sit in a dark room with: _____

The best part of my day: _____

Something that made me laugh: _____

Whom did I let "off the hook" today? _____

Someone / Something that brings me joy: _____

Where kindness touched my world today: _____

How I nourished my mind, body or spirit: _____

Number of hours I rested or slept in past 24 hours:
___ Rest   ___ Sleep

Prayer/Meditation for the day:
☼ Yes   ☼ No

I am grateful for: _____

Today I did this one little thing
    For the earth...
        for a friend or a stranger...
           for someone older or younger...
              for someone sicker...
                in more need... _____

November 16TH

Someone I value: _____

The best part of my day: _____

Something that made me laugh: _____

Whom did I let "off the hook" today? _____

Someone / Something that brings me joy: _____

Where kindness touched my world today: _____

How I nourished my mind, body or spirit: _____

Number of hours I rested or slept in past 24 hours:
____ Rest   ____ Sleep

Prayer/Meditation for the day:
☼ Yes   ☼ No

I am grateful for: _____

Today I did this one little thing
    For the earth...
        for a friend or a stranger...
            for someone older or younger...
                for someone sicker...
                    in more need... _____

> " *We all must try to be the best person we can by making the best choices and by making the most of the talents we've been given.* "
> —MARY LOU RETTON

A talent I try to make the most of: _____

The best part of my day: _____

Something that made me laugh: _____

Whom did I let "off the hook" today? _____

Someone / Something that brings me joy: _____

Where kindness touched my world today: _____

How I nourished my mind, body or spirit: _____

Number of hours I rested or slept in past 24 hours:
___ Rest ___ Sleep

Prayer/Meditation for the day:
☼ Yes ☼ No

I am grateful for: _____

Today I did this one little thing
    For the earth...
        for a friend or a stranger...
            for someone older or younger...
                for someone sicker...
                    in more need... _____

November 18TH

> " *Do not avoid DOING life because you might have to go find a place to rest halfway through some event. It's better to do something half-way, and enjoy those minutes, than to do nothing 100%.* "
> —JACQUE MCFARLAND

I want to feel: _____

The best part of my day: _____

Something that made me laugh: _____

Whom did I let "off the hook" today? _____

Someone / Something that brings me joy: _____

Where kindness touched my world today: _____

How I nourished my mind, body or spirit: _____

Number of hours I rested or slept in past 24 hours:
____ Rest ____ Sleep

Prayer/Meditation for the day:
☼ Yes ☼ No

I am grateful for: _____

Today I did this one little thing
    For the earth...
        for a friend or a stranger...
            for someone older or younger...
                for someone sicker...
                    in more need... _____

> " *You gain strength, courage, and confidence by every experience in which you really stop to look fear in the face. You are able to say to yourself, "I have lived through this horror. I can take the next thing that comes along." You must do the thing you think you cannot do.* "
> —ELEANOR ROOSEVELT

Something devastating that I have
overcome and how it has changed me: _____

The best part of my day: _____

Something that made me laugh: _____

Whom did I let "off the hook" today? _____

Someone / Something that brings me joy: _____

Where kindness touched my world today: _____

How I nourished my mind, body or spirit: _____

Number of hours I rested or slept in past 24 hours:
___ Rest ___ Sleep

Prayer/Meditation for the day:
☼ Yes ☼ No

I am grateful for: _____

Today I did this one little thing
    For the earth...
        for a friend or a stranger...
            for someone older or younger...
                for someone sicker...
                    in more need... _____

November 20TH

" In and out up and down over and over she wove her strands of life together.
patching hole after hole eventually; she saw it was more than the threads that
gave her strength, it was in the very act of weaving itself, that she became strong. "

—TERRI ST. CLOUD
BONESIGHARTS.COM

My strength comes from: _____

The best part of my day: _____

Something that made me laugh: _____

Whom did I let "off the hook" today? _____

Someone / Something that brings me joy: _____

Where kindness touched my world today: _____

How I nourished my mind, body or spirit: _____

Number of hours I rested or slept in past 24 hours:
____ Rest   ____ Sleep

Prayer/Meditation for the day:
☼ Yes   ☼ No

I am grateful for: _____

Today I did this one little thing
    For the earth...
        for a friend or a stranger...
            for someone older or younger...
                for someone sicker...
                    in more need... _____

10 Day Overview

Best part of the past ten days? _____

Number of days I laughed: _____

Goal I want to set for the next 10 days: _____

Person/people who did or
said something to help me heal: _____

Anything else I have noticed
or want to remember/record: _____

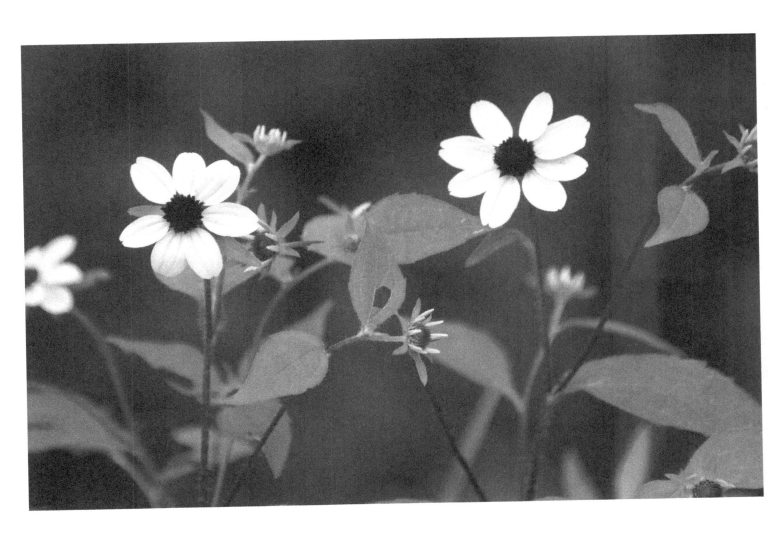

November 21ST

> *"You learn the most about yourself from teaching and sharing with others."*
> —KATHRYN STARKE

Whom did I share with today? _____

The best part of my day: _____

Something that made me laugh: _____

Whom did I let "off the hook" today? _____

Someone / Something that brings me joy: _____

Where kindness touched my world today: _____

How I nourished my mind, body or spirit: _____

Number of hours I rested or slept in past 24 hours:
___ Rest ___ Sleep

Prayer/Meditation for the day:
☼ Yes ☼ No

I am grateful for: _____

Today I did this one little thing
    For the earth...
        for a friend or a stranger...
           for someone older or younger...
              for someone sicker...
                in more need... _____

November 22ND

" We don't always have to know why. Spending too much time
on the why takes away from figuring out what to do next. "
—SANDRA BECK

How has/does spending too much
time asking "why" affect my healing? _____

The best part of my day: _____

Something that made me laugh: _____

Whom did I let "off the hook" today? _____

Someone / Something that brings me joy: _____

Where kindness touched my world today: _____

How I nourished my mind, body or spirit: _____

Number of hours I rested or slept in past 24 hours:
___Rest   ___Sleep

Prayer/Meditation for the day:
☼ Yes   ☼ No

I am grateful for: _____

Today I did this one little thing
   For the earth...
      for a friend or a stranger...
         for someone older or younger...
            for someone sicker...
               in more need... _____

November 23RD

> *"Life's under no obligation to give us what we expect. We take what we get and are thankful it's no worse than it is."*
> —MARGARET MITCHELL

What am I thankful of that it is no worse: _____

The best part of my day: _____

Something that made me laugh: _____

Whom did I let "off the hook" today? _____

Someone / Something that brings me joy: _____

Where kindness touched my world today: _____

How I nourished my mind, body or spirit: _____

Number of hours I rested or slept in past 24 hours:
___ Rest   ___ Sleep

Prayer/Meditation for the day:
☼ Yes   ☼ No

I am grateful for: _____

Today I did this one little thing
    For the earth...
        for a friend or a stranger...
            for someone older or younger...
                for someone sicker...
                    in more need... _____

> *"What I have found through a tumultuous and difficult*
> *early life is that acceptance is the road to freedom."*
> —DAVID PATTEN

What have I learned to accept? _____

The best part of my day: _____

Something that made me laugh: _____

Whom did I let "off the hook" today? _____

Someone / Something that brings me joy: _____

Where kindness touched my world today: _____

How I nourished my mind, body or spirit: _____

Number of hours I rested or slept in past 24 hours:
___Rest ___Sleep

Prayer/Meditation for the day:
☼ Yes ☼ No

I am grateful for: _____

Today I did this one little thing
    For the earth...
        for a friend or a stranger...
           for someone older or younger...
              for someone sicker...
                in more need... _____

November 25TH

"Happiness is not a possession to be prized, it is a quality of thought, a state of mind."
—DAPHNE DU MAURIER

What quality do I most want
to share with the world? _____

The best part of my day: _____

Something that made me laugh: _____

Whom did I let "off the hook" today? _____

Someone / Something that brings me joy: _____

Where kindness touched my world today: _____

How I nourished my mind, body or spirit: _____

Number of hours I rested or slept in past 24 hours:
___Rest   ___Sleep

Prayer/Meditation for the day:
☼ Yes   ☼ No

I am grateful for: _____

Today I did this one little thing
    For the earth...
        for a friend or a stranger...
           for someone older or younger...
               for someone sicker...
                   in more need... _____

November 26TH

"I am proud of the scars in my soul. They remind me that I have an intense life."
—PAULO COELHO

What scar am I proud of? _____

The best part of my day: _____

Something that made me laugh: _____

Whom did I let "off the hook" today? _____

Someone / Something that brings me joy: _____

Where kindness touched my world today: _____

How I nourished my mind, body or spirit: _____

Number of hours I rested or slept in past 24 hours:
___Rest   ___Sleep

Prayer/Meditation for the day:
☼ Yes   ☼ No

I am grateful for: _____

Today I did this one little thing
    For the earth...
        for a friend or a stranger...
           for someone older or younger...
              for someone sicker...
                in more need... _____

November 27TH

" *The greatest part of our happiness depends on our dispositions, not our circumstances.* **"**
—MARTHA WASHINGTON

What type of attitude did I have today? _____

The best part of my day: _____

Something that made me laugh: _____

Whom did I let "off the hook" today? _____

Someone / Something that brings me joy: _____

Where kindness touched my world today: _____

How I nourished my mind, body or spirit: _____

Number of hours I rested or slept in past 24 hours:
___Rest ___Sleep

Prayer/Meditation for the day:
☼ Yes ☼ No

I am grateful for: _____

Today I did this one little thing
    For the earth...
        for a friend or a stranger...
            for someone older or younger...
                for someone sicker...
                    in more need... _____

" How do you want to say goodbye?"
— SHARON RAINEY

The best way someone said goodbye to me: _____

The best part of my day: _____

Something that made me laugh: _____

Whom did I let "off the hook" today? _____

Someone / Something that brings me joy: _____

Where kindness touched my world today: _____

How I nourished my mind, body or spirit: _____

Number of hours I rested or slept in past 24 hours:
___ Rest ___ Sleep

Prayer/Meditation for the day:
☼ Yes ☼ No

I am grateful for: _____

Today I did this one little thing
    For the earth...
        for a friend or a stranger...
            for someone older or younger...
                for someone sicker...
                    in more need... _____

November 29th

*"One of the most courageous things you can do is identify yourself,
know who you are, what you believe in and where you want to go."*
—SHEILA MURRAY BETHEL

What do I believe? Where do I want to go? _____

The best part of my day: _____

Something that made me laugh: _____

Whom did I let "off the hook" today? _____

Someone / Something that brings me joy: _____

Where kindness touched my world today: _____

How I nourished my mind, body or spirit: _____

Number of hours I rested or slept in past 24 hours:
___ Rest   ___ Sleep

Prayer/Meditation for the day:
☼ Yes   ☼ No

I am grateful for: _____

Today I did this one little thing
    For the earth...
        for a friend or a stranger...
            for someone older or younger...
                for someone sicker...
                    in more need... _____

" In this life we cannot always do great things,
but we can do small things with great love."
—MOTHER TERESA

What I did today with great love: _____

The best part of my day: _____

Something that made me laugh: _____

Whom did I let "off the hook" today? _____

Someone / Something that brings me joy: _____

Where kindness touched my world today: _____

How I nourished my mind, body or spirit: _____

Number of hours I rested or slept in past 24 hours:
___ Rest ___ Sleep

Prayer/Meditation for the day:
☼ Yes ☼ No

I am grateful for: _____

Today I did this one little thing
    For the earth...
        for a friend or a stranger...
           for someone older or younger...
             for someone sicker...
                in more need... _____

End of Month Review

Best part of the past ten days? _____

Number of days I laughed: _____

Goal I want to set for the next 10 days: _____

Person/people who did or
said something to help me heal: _____

Anything else I have noticed
or want to remember/record: _____

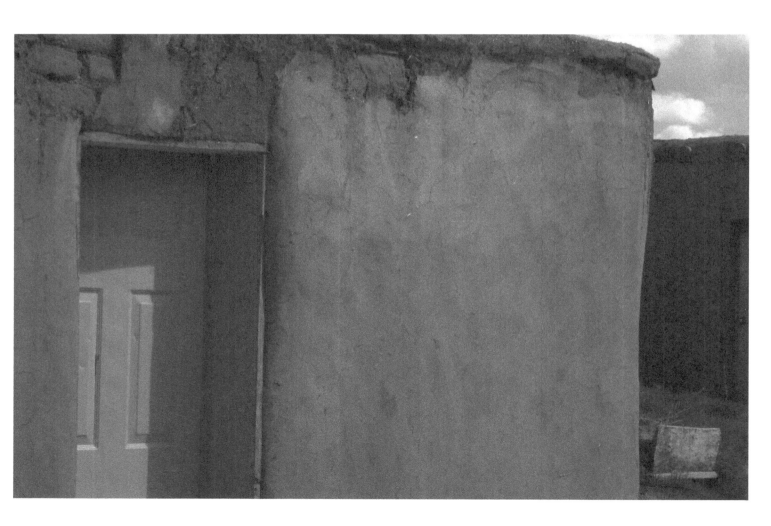

" *You cannot hate, argue, reason, fight, complain or yell at a dark room enough to illuminate it - only by shining a light is darkness overcome. Be that light.* "
—ANONYMOUS

The light that I shine… _____

The best part of my day: _____

Something that made me laugh: _____

Whom did I let "off the hook" today? _____

Someone / Something that brings me joy: _____

Where kindness touched my world today: _____

How I nourished my mind, body or spirit: _____

Number of hours I rested or slept in past 24 hours:
___ Rest ___ Sleep

Prayer/Meditation for the day:
☼ Yes ☼ No

I am grateful for: _____

Today I did this one little thing
    For the earth…
        for a friend or a stranger…
            for someone older or younger…
                for someone sicker…
                    in more need… _____

December 2ND

"Hate is too great a burden to bear. It injures the hater more than it injures the hated."
—CORETTA SCOTT KING

Where have I let go of the hate? _____

The best part of my day: _____

Something that made me laugh: _____

Whom did I let "off the hook" today? _____

Someone / Something that brings me joy: _____

Where kindness touched my world today: _____

How I nourished my mind, body or spirit: _____

Number of hours I rested or slept in past 24 hours:
___ Rest ___ Sleep

Prayer/Meditation for the day:
☀ Yes ☀ No

I am grateful for: _____

Today I did this one little thing
    For the earth...
        for a friend or a stranger...
            for someone older or younger...
                for someone sicker...
                    in more need... _____

" You block your dream when you allow your fear to grow bigger than your faith. "
—MARY MANIN MORRISSEY

What dream do I want to encourage today? _____

The best part of my day: _____

Something that made me laugh: _____

Whom did I let "off the hook" today? _____

Someone / Something that brings me joy: _____

Where kindness touched my world today: _____

How I nourished my mind, body or spirit: _____

Number of hours I rested or slept in past 24 hours:
___Rest ___Sleep

Prayer/Meditation for the day:
☼ Yes ☼ No

I am grateful for: _____

Today I did this one little thing
    For the earth...
        for a friend or a stranger...
           for someone older or younger...
              for someone sicker...
                in more need... _____

December 4TH

"What anyone else has or does not have has nothing to do with you. The only thing that affects your experience is the way you utilize the Non-Physical Energy with your thought. Your abundance or lack of it in your experience has nothing to do with what anybody else is doing or having. It has only to do with your perspective. It has only to do with your offering of thought. If you want your fortunes to shift, you have to begin telling a different story."

—ESTHER ABRAHAM-HICKS

MONEY, AND THE LAW OF ATTRACTION: LEARNING TO ATTRACT WEALTH, HEALTH, AND HAPPINESS

How I have started to tell a different story: _____

The best part of my day: _____

Something that made me laugh: _____

Whom did I let "off the hook" today? _____

Someone / Something that brings me joy: _____

Where kindness touched my world today: _____

How I nourished my mind, body or spirit: _____

Number of hours I rested or slept in past 24 hours:
___ Rest   ___ Sleep

Prayer/Meditation for the day:
☼ Yes   ☼ No

I am grateful for: _____

Today I did this one little thing
    For the earth...
        for a friend or a stranger...
            for someone older or younger...
                for someone sicker...
                    in more need... _____

*"I may not have gone where I intended to go, but
I think I have ended up where I needed to be."*
—DOUGLAS ADAMS

How I know I am where I need to be: _____

The best part of my day: _____

Something that made me laugh: _____

Whom did I let "off the hook" today? _____

Someone / Something that brings me joy: _____

Where kindness touched my world today: _____

How I nourished my mind, body or spirit: _____

Number of hours I rested or slept in past 24 hours:
___ Rest ___ Sleep

Prayer/Meditation for the day:
☼ Yes   ☼ No

I am grateful for: _____

Today I did this one little thing
    For the earth...
        for a friend or a stranger...
            for someone older or younger...
                for someone sicker...
                    in more need... _____

December 6TH

"Love is a fruit in season at all times and within reach of every hand."
—MOTHER TERESA

Where/How I saw Love today: _____

The best part of my day: _____

Something that made me laugh: _____

Whom did I let "off the hook" today? _____

Someone / Something that brings me joy: _____

Where kindness touched my world today: _____

How I nourished my mind, body or spirit: _____

Number of hours I rested or slept in past 24 hours:
___ Rest   ___ Sleep

Prayer/Meditation for the day:
☼ Yes   ☼ No

I am grateful for: _____

Today I did this one little thing
    For the earth...
        for a friend or a stranger...
            for someone older or younger...
                for someone sicker...
                    in more need... _____

December 7TH

> " *There are no shortcuts through the seasons. Each holds its own challenges, and gifts. Be present and appreciative of the lessons through it all, for the joy fades as surely as the sorrow.* "
> —LYNDA DAVIS

When have I wanted to give up? What have
I gained from not giving up in the past? _____

The best part of my day: _____

Something that made me laugh: _____

Whom did I let "off the hook" today? _____

Someone / Something that brings me joy: _____

Where kindness touched my world today: _____

How I nourished my mind, body or spirit: _____

Number of hours I rested or slept in past 24 hours:
___Rest ___Sleep

Prayer/Meditation for the day:
☼ Yes ☼ No

I am grateful for: _____

Today I did this one little thing
    For the earth...
        for a friend or a stranger...
           for someone older or younger...
             for someone sicker...
                in more need... _____

December 8TH

> " *I suspect the truth is that we are waiting, all of us, against insurmountable odds, for something extraordinary to happen to us.* "
> —KHALED HOSSEINI
> *AND THE MOUNTAINS ECHOED*

When have I wanted to give up? What have
I gained from not giving up in the past? _____

The best part of my day: _____

Something that made me laugh: _____

Whom did I let "off the hook" today? _____

Someone / Something that brings me joy: _____

Where kindness touched my world today: _____

How I nourished my mind, body or spirit: _____

Number of hours I rested or slept in past 24 hours:
___Rest   ___Sleep

Prayer/Meditation for the day:
☼ Yes   ☼ No

I am grateful for: _____

Today I did this one little thing
    For the earth...
        for a friend or a stranger...
            for someone older or younger...
                for someone sicker...
                    in more need... _____

December 9TH

> **"***The power of intention came to be recognized as an important critical factor in catalyzing potentiality and actuality.***"**
>
> —DAVID HAWKINS, MD
> *HEALING AND RECOVERY*

One of my intentions is: _____

The best part of my day: _____

Something that made me laugh: _____

Whom did I let "off the hook" today? _____

Someone / Something that brings me joy: _____

Where kindness touched my world today: _____

How I nourished my mind, body or spirit: _____

Number of hours I rested or slept in past 24 hours:
___Rest   ___Sleep

Prayer/Meditation for the day:
☼ Yes   ☼ No

I am grateful for: _____

Today I did this one little thing
    For the earth...
        for a friend or a stranger...
           for someone older or younger...
               for someone sicker...
                  in more need... _____

December 10TH

"When illness is part of your spiritual journey, no medical intervention can heal you until your spirit has begun to make the necessary changes that the illness was designed to inspire."
—CAROLINE MYSS

One way I have started to heal spiritually: _____

The best part of my day: _____

Something that made me laugh: _____

Whom did I let "off the hook" today? _____

Someone / Something that brings me joy: _____

Where kindness touched my world today: _____

How I nourished my mind, body or spirit: _____

Number of hours I rested or slept in past 24 hours:
___ Rest ___ Sleep

Prayer/Meditation for the day:
☼ Yes ☼ No

I am grateful for: _____

Today I did this one little thing
    For the earth...
        for a friend or a stranger...
            for someone older or younger...
               for someone sicker...
                  in more need... _____

Early Month Review

Best part of the past ten days? _____

Number of days I laughed: _____

Goal I want to set for the next 10 days: _____

Person/people who did or
said something to help me heal: _____

Anything else I have noticed
or want to remember/record: _____

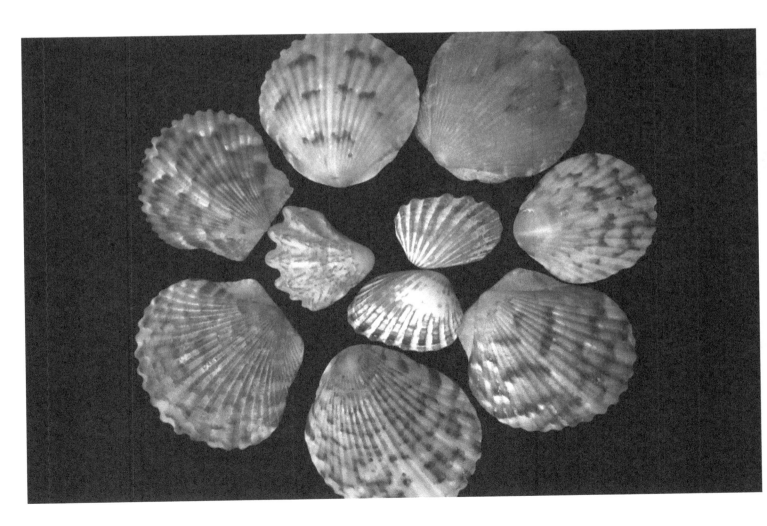

December 11TH

> *" What and how much had I lost by trying to do only what was expected of me instead of what I myself had wished to do?"*
>
> —RALPH ELLISON

What I wish, what I want to do: _____

The best part of my day: _____

Something that made me laugh: _____

Whom did I let "off the hook" today? _____

Someone / Something that brings me joy: _____

Where kindness touched my world today: _____

How I nourished my mind, body or spirit: _____

Number of hours I rested or slept in past 24 hours:
___ Rest   ___ Sleep

Prayer/Meditation for the day:
☼ Yes   ☼ No

I am grateful for: _____

Today I did this one little thing
    For the earth...
        for a friend or a stranger...
            for someone older or younger...
                for someone sicker...
                    in more need... _____

December 12TH

> **"***Let the spirit tell the body what to do because if you let
> the body tell the spirit what to do, nothing will get done.***"**
> —UNDERCOVER BOSS

What is my body telling me to do?
What would happen if I listened? _____

The best part of my day: _____

Something that made me laugh: _____

Whom did I let "off the hook" today? _____

Someone / Something that brings me joy: _____

Where kindness touched my world today: _____

How I nourished my mind, body or spirit: _____

Number of hours I rested or slept in past 24 hours:
___Rest ___Sleep

Prayer/Meditation for the day:
☀ Yes ☀ No

I am grateful for: _____

Today I did this one little thing
　　For the earth...
　　　　for a friend or a stranger...
　　　　　　for someone older or younger...
　　　　　　　　for someone sicker...
　　　　　　　　　　in more need... _____

December 13TH

"It's not how hard you hit. It's how hard you get hit... and keep moving forward."

—RANDY PAUSCH

I have been hit hard by _____ but
keep moving forward.

The best part of my day: _____

Something that made me laugh: _____

Whom did I let "off the hook" today? _____

Someone / Something that brings me joy: _____

Where kindness touched my world today: _____

How I nourished my mind, body or spirit: _____

Number of hours I rested or slept in past 24 hours:
___ Rest   ___ Sleep

Prayer/Meditation for the day:
☼ Yes   ☼ No

I am grateful for: _____

Today I did this one little thing
    For the earth...
        for a friend or a stranger...
            for someone older or younger...
                for someone sicker...
                    in more need... _____

" It is not who you are that holds you back; it's who you think you are not. "
—DENIS WAITLEY

Am I focusing on the part of
what I am or what I am not? _____

The best part of my day: _____

Something that made me laugh: _____

Whom did I let "off the hook" today? _____

Someone / Something that brings me joy: _____

Where kindness touched my world today: _____

How I nourished my mind, body or spirit: _____

Number of hours I rested or slept in past 24 hours:
___ Rest ___ Sleep

Prayer/Meditation for the day:
☼ Yes ☼ No

I am grateful for: _____

Today I did this one little thing
    For the earth...
        for a friend or a stranger...
            for someone older or younger...
                for someone sicker...
                    in more need... _____

December 15TH

> "*I don't Fight this disease. I do Fight for Healing. I Fight for Hope. I try to make Peace with this Journey. I have Overcome so much before so many times, and this will be another.*"
> —ALISA TURNER

What word resonates with me today?
⁙ Fight ⁙ Heal ⁙ Hope
⁙ Peace ⁙ Journey ⁙ Overcome

The best part of my day: _____

Something that made me laugh: _____

Whom did I let "off the hook" today? _____

Someone / Something that brings me joy: _____

Where kindness touched my world today: _____

How I nourished my mind, body or spirit: _____

Number of hours I rested or slept in past 24 hours:
___ Rest ___ Sleep

Prayer/Meditation for the day:
⁙ Yes ⁙ No

I am grateful for: _____

Today I did this one little thing
   For the earth...
      for a friend or a stranger...
         for someone older or younger...
           for someone sicker...
              in more need... _____

"*The clouds were building up now for the trade wind and he looked ahead and saw a flight of wild ducks etching themselves against the sky over the water, then blurring, then etching again and he knew no man was ever alone on the sea.*"
—ERNEST HEMINGWAY

Someone who flew over, letting
me know I am not alone: _____

The best part of my day: _____

Something that made me laugh: _____

Whom did I let "off the hook" today? _____

Someone / Something that brings me joy: _____

Where kindness touched my world today: _____

How I nourished my mind, body or spirit: _____

Number of hours I rested or slept in past 24 hours:
___ Rest ___ Sleep

Prayer/Meditation for the day:
☼ Yes ☼ No

I am grateful for: _____

Today I did this one little thing
  For the earth...
    for a friend or a stranger...
      for someone older or younger...
        for someone sicker...
          in more need... _____

December 17TH

"In grief, the world looks poor and empty. In depression, the person feels poor and empty."
—SIGMUND FREUD

Where I saw fullness and wealth today: _____

The best part of my day: _____

Something that made me laugh: _____

Whom did I let "off the hook" today? _____

Someone / Something that brings me joy: _____

Where kindness touched my world today: _____

How I nourished my mind, body or spirit: _____

Number of hours I rested or slept in past 24 hours:
___ Rest   ___ Sleep

Prayer/Meditation for the day:
☼ Yes   ☼ No

I am grateful for: _____

Today I did this one little thing
    For the earth...
        for a friend or a stranger...
           for someone older or younger...
               for someone sicker...
                  in more need... _____

"*You must give up the life you planned in order to have the life that is waiting for you.*"
—JOSEPH CAMPBELL

Am I accepting of my life as it is today? _____

The best part of my day: _____

Something that made me laugh: _____

Whom did I let "off the hook" today? _____

Someone / Something that brings me joy: _____

Where kindness touched my world today: _____

How I nourished my mind, body or spirit: _____

Number of hours I rested or slept in past 24 hours:
___ Rest ___ Sleep

Prayer/Meditation for the day:
☼ Yes ☼ No

I am grateful for: _____

Today I did this one little thing
  For the earth...
    for a friend or a stranger...
      for someone older or younger...
        for someone sicker...
          in more need... _____

December 19th

"If you cannot be thankful for what you have received, be thankful for what you have escaped."
—AMISH PROVERB

I am grateful for: _____

The best part of my day: _____

Something that made me laugh: _____

Whom did I let "off the hook" today? _____

Someone / Something that brings me joy: _____

Where kindness touched my world today: _____

How I nourished my mind, body or spirit: _____

Number of hours I rested or slept in past 24 hours:
___ Rest   ___ Sleep

Prayer/Meditation for the day:
☼ Yes   ☼ No

I am grateful for: _____

Today I did this one little thing
    For the earth...
        for a friend or a stranger...
           for someone older or younger...
               for someone sicker...
                  in more need... _____

December 20TH

"We will have to repent in this generation not merely for the vitriolic words and actions of the bad people, but for the appalling silence of the good people."
—MARTIN LUTHER KING, JR.

I choose not to be silent about: _____

The best part of my day: _____

Something that made me laugh: _____

Whom did I let "off the hook" today? _____

Someone / Something that brings me joy: _____

Where kindness touched my world today: _____

How I nourished my mind, body or spirit: _____

Number of hours I rested or slept in past 24 hours:
___ Rest ___ Sleep

Prayer/Meditation for the day:
☼ Yes   ☼ No

I am grateful for: _____

Today I did this one little thing
    For the earth...
        for a friend or a stranger...
            for someone older or younger...
                for someone sicker...
                    in more need... _____

Mid Month
Review

Best part of the past ten days? _____

Number of days I laughed: _____

Goal I want to set for the next 10 days: _____

Person/people who did or
said something to help me heal: _____

Anything else I have noticed
or want to remember/record: _____

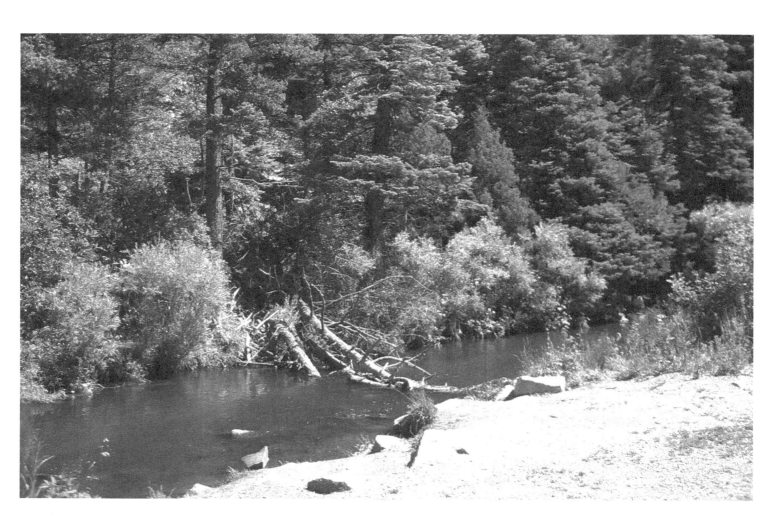

> **"** *You have enemies? Good. That means you've*
> *stood up for something, sometime in your life.* **"**
> —WINSTON CHURCHILL

Something I recently stood up for: _____

The best part of my day: _____

Something that made me laugh: _____

Whom did I let "off the hook" today? _____

Someone / Something that brings me joy: _____

Where kindness touched my world today: _____

How I nourished my mind, body or spirit: _____

Number of hours I rested or slept in past 24 hours:
____Rest   ____Sleep

Prayer/Meditation for the day:
☼ Yes   ☼ No

I am grateful for: _____

Today I did this one little thing
    For the earth...
        for a friend or a stranger...
            for someone older or younger...
                for someone sicker...
                    in more need... _____

December 22ND

> "*Reflect upon your present blessings, of which every man has many; not on your past misfortunes, of which all men have some.*"
> —CHARLES DICKENS

Five of my greatest blessings: _____

The best part of my day: _____

Something that made me laugh: _____

Whom did I let "off the hook" today? _____

Someone / Something that brings me joy: _____

Where kindness touched my world today: _____

How I nourished my mind, body or spirit: _____

Number of hours I rested or slept in past 24 hours:
___Rest   ___Sleep

Prayer/Meditation for the day:
☼ Yes   ☼ No

I am grateful for: _____

Today I did this one little thing
    For the earth...
        for a friend or a stranger...
            for someone older or younger...
                for someone sicker...
                    in more need... _____

> " *Cherish your visions and your dreams as they are the children of your soul, the blueprints of your ultimate achievements.* "
> —NAPOLEON HILL

One of my dreams/visions: _____

The best part of my day: _____

Something that made me laugh: _____

Whom did I let "off the hook" today? _____

Someone / Something that brings me joy: _____

Where kindness touched my world today: _____

How I nourished my mind, body or spirit: _____

Number of hours I rested or slept in past 24 hours:
___Rest   ___Sleep

Prayer/Meditation for the day:
☼ Yes   ☼ No

I am grateful for: _____

Today I did this one little thing
   For the earth...
      for a friend or a stranger...
         for someone older or younger...
            for someone sicker...
               in more need... _____

December 24TH

"*Love is the answer; the question doesn't matter.*"
—DR. BERNIE SIEGEL

A time when love was truly the right answer: _____

The best part of my day: _____

Something that made me laugh: _____

Whom did I let "off the hook" today? _____

Someone / Something that brings me joy: _____

Where kindness touched my world today: _____

How I nourished my mind, body or spirit: _____

Number of hours I rested or slept in past 24 hours:
___ Rest ___ Sleep

Prayer/Meditation for the day:
☼ Yes ☼ No

I am grateful for: _____

Today I did this one little thing
    For the earth...
        for a friend or a stranger...
            for someone older or younger...
                for someone sicker...
                    in more need... _____

" *A real decision is measured by the fact that you've taken a new action. If there's no action, you haven't truly decided.* "
—TONY ROBBINS

A decision that I have acted upon: _____

The best part of my day: _____

Something that made me laugh: _____

Whom did I let "off the hook" today? _____

Someone / Something that brings me joy: _____

Where kindness touched my world today: _____

How I nourished my mind, body or spirit: _____

Number of hours I rested or slept in past 24 hours:
___Rest   ___Sleep

Prayer/Meditation for the day:
☼ Yes   ☼ No

I am grateful for: _____

Today I did this one little thing
    For the earth...
        for a friend or a stranger...
            for someone older or younger...
                for someone sicker...
                    in more need... _____

December 26TH

"A mediocre person tells. A good person explains. A superior person demonstrates. A great person inspires others to see for themselves."
—HARVEY MACKAY

Whom have I inspired? Or
how have I inspired others? _____

The best part of my day: _____

Something that made me laugh: _____

Whom did I let "off the hook" today? _____

Someone / Something that brings me joy: _____

Where kindness touched my world today: _____

How I nourished my mind, body or spirit: _____

Number of hours I rested or slept in past 24 hours:
___ Rest ___ Sleep

Prayer/Meditation for the day:
☼ Yes ☼ No

I am grateful for: _____

Today I did this one little thing
    For the earth...
        for a friend or a stranger...
            for someone older or younger...
                for someone sicker...
                    in more need... _____

December 27TH

"I am more than my physical body. This simple acknowledgment has profound implications."
—ROBERT MONROE

One of the best qualities of my soul is: _____

The best part of my day: _____

Something that made me laugh: _____

Whom did I let "off the hook" today? _____

Someone / Something that brings me joy: _____

Where kindness touched my world today: _____

How I nourished my mind, body or spirit: _____

Number of hours I rested or slept in past 24 hours:
___Rest ___Sleep

Prayer/Meditation for the day:
☼ Yes   ☼ No

I am grateful for: _____

Today I did this one little thing
　　For the earth...
　　　　for a friend or a stranger...
　　　　　　for someone older or younger...
　　　　　　　　for someone sicker...
　　　　　　　　　　in more need... _____

December 28TH

"Raise your acceptance; lower your expectations."
—SHARON RAINEY

What can I be more accepting of? _____

The best part of my day: _____

Something that made me laugh: _____

Whom did I let "off the hook" today? _____

Someone / Something that brings me joy: _____

Where kindness touched my world today: _____

How I nourished my mind, body or spirit: _____

Number of hours I rested or slept in past 24 hours:
___ Rest ___ Sleep

Prayer/Meditation for the day:
☼ Yes ☼ No

I am grateful for: _____

Today I did this one little thing
   For the earth...
      for a friend or a stranger...
         for someone older or younger...
           for someone sicker...
              in more need... _____

" The best time to plant a tree was 20 years ago. The second best time is now. "
—CHINESE PROVERB

What can I do today that
will help me in the future? _____

The best part of my day: _____

Something that made me laugh: _____

Whom did I let "off the hook" today? _____

Someone / Something that brings me joy: _____

Where kindness touched my world today: _____

How I nourished my mind, body or spirit: _____

Number of hours I rested or slept in past 24 hours:
___Rest ___Sleep

Prayer/Meditation for the day:
☼ Yes ☼ No

I am grateful for: _____

Today I did this one little thing
   For the earth...
      for a friend or a stranger...
         for someone older or younger...
           for someone sicker...
              in more need... _____

December 30TH

"*Hope is a song in a weary throat.***"**
—PAULI MURRAY

The song that I sung when I was hopeless: _____

The best part of my day: _____

Something that made me laugh: _____

Whom did I let "off the hook" today? _____

Someone / Something that brings me joy: _____

Where kindness touched my world today: _____

How I nourished my mind, body or spirit: _____

Number of hours I rested or slept in past 24 hours:
___ Rest ___ Sleep

Prayer/Meditation for the day:
☼ Yes ☼ No

I am grateful for: _____

Today I did this one little thing
    For the earth...
        for a friend or a stranger...
            for someone older or younger...
                for someone sicker...
                    in more need... _____

December 31ST

> **"*Attention energizes; intention transforms.*"**
> —SHARON RAINEY

I intend to: _____

The best part of my day: _____

Something that made me laugh: _____

Whom did I let "off the hook" today? _____

Someone / Something that brings me joy: _____

Where kindness touched my world today: _____

How I nourished my mind, body or spirit: _____

Number of hours I rested or slept in past 24 hours:
____Rest ____Sleep

Prayer/Meditation for the day:
☼ Yes ☼ No

I am grateful for: _____

Today I did this one little thing
    For the earth...
        for a friend or a stranger...
           for someone older or younger...
              for someone sicker...
                in more need... _____

End of Month Review

Best part of the past ten days? _____

Number of days I laughed: _____

Goal I want to set for the next 10 days: _____

Person/people who did or
said something to help me heal: _____

Anything else I have noticed
or want to remember/record: _____

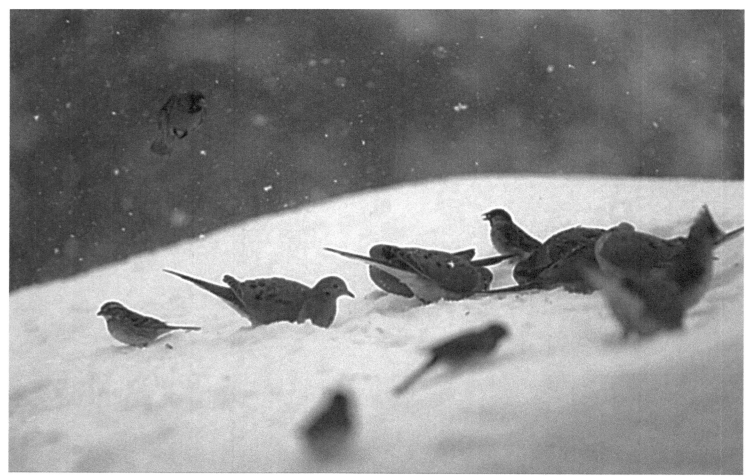

©JOE KELLY

I am from

The Source

Lover of Light and Laughter

I am from dancing and playing Angels and petulant Souls

I am from Priests

Assigned Sacred Tasks

I collect the sacred tears, the profound sadness

Offering alms.

I am from a groovy, magical, mysterious pink waiting room

filled with fresh blossoms and sunlight.

I am from vast Grand Canyon abstract landscapes,

deep as the suffering in your soul.

I am from Blue eyes and Green eyes and Brown eyes.

I am from Eyes that see only my Soul and Hearts that love me with all.

I am a Channel, a Translator, a part of and sometimes a part from

I am Connected and Isolated instantly and eternally

I am from what was, what is, what cannot and yet will be.

I am from grey Dust, emerald Gems.

I write,

I sing, I suffer,

I wonder, I wander

I heal and I return

All in Love.

SHARON E. RAINEY

(2.18.16)

Acknowledgements

Mom and Dad (Earle and June Williams) – my life today is as it is because of your generosity, your kind spirit and infinite love for your children and grandchildren; **Jeff Rainey** – the depth and breadth of your love for me remain my bedrock. Your acceptance of my very imperfect self fascinate and comfort me. When you reach for my hand and reassure me that we will hurdle the next obstacle together, I am humbled and even more grateful; **Heather Rainey** – your choices in life, in education, in work, and in love demonstrate the depth of healing you have achieved. Thank you for allowing me to share in your journey and to remain an integral part of your life. Every day, you walk the walk and I am enamored by your dedication and determination; **Joey Rainey** – I love you. And I will always love you; **Stephen Rainey** – Thank you for turning the question around and asking me about my own Best Parts of the Day. This book may never have been written had you not done so; **Robert Mozayeni** – thank you for your courage and diligence in asking me the hard questions, tenacity in learning the intricacies of my diseases, sharing your own journey with me, and for healing my body; **Beth Renne** – thank you for the reflections, the insights, the encouragement, the foresight, the compassion; **Joanne Muir** – your energy encourages and reassures me, your smile comforts me. Thank you for holding my vulnerability sacred; **Suzanne Mozayeni** – thank you for challenging me to meditate. The path was long, but you led me to the place I needed to be; **the hundreds of friends in 12 Step Recovery programs** – thank you for your willingness to love me until I could love myself, for your willingness to share your healing journeys with me; **the Saturday group 'meeting after the meeting'** – the intimacy we share through horrible and uncertain times is like no other I have anywhere else. I am honored to be witness to each chapter that our respective lives write; **MB @zebrafinch** – thank you for accepting my love, for letting me say I Love You every time we talk; **Deb Jansen** - thank you for teaching me to laugh at it all; to see the absurdity, the beauty, the determination to find the answer; thank you for showing me the Art of Living, Loving, and Laughing; **Robin Shirley** – the light of your soul shimmers as you share with others your encouragement, insight, and love of simplicity. Your acts of kindness helped quicken my own healing; **Gary Glaser** – RIP, brother. Your kindness and generosity were always a better part of each day for me; **Alyssa Knapp** – your smile, twisted humor, optimism, and determination align me with my own healing path; **the thousands of chronically ill patients** – even with the multiple setbacks we all encounter, for showing and sharing with me what works and what needs tweaking, for showing me the joy, the healing, and the success.